THROUGH
the VALLEYS

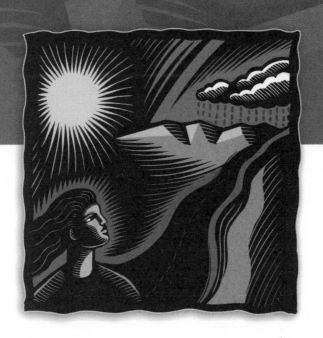

Finding Triumph in the Trials of Life

THROUGH the VALLEYS

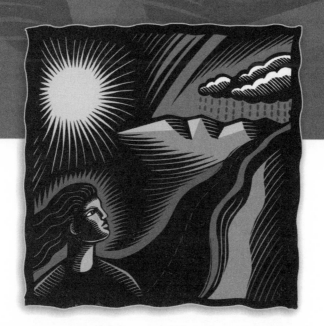

ERNEST L. EASLEY

BROADMAN
& HOLMAN
PUBLISHERS

NASHVILLE, TENNESSEE

0–8054–3199–3

Published by Broadman & Holman Publishers
Nashville, Tennessee

Dewey Decimal Classification: 242
Subject Heading: DEVOTIONAL LITERATURE \
CHRISTIAN LIFE \ JOY AND SORROW

Scripture quotations are from the New King James Version,
copyright © 1979, 1980, 1982, Thomas Nelson, Inc., Publishers.
Italic type in Scripture text has sometimes been added
for emphasis.

1 2 3 4 5 6 7 8 9 10 10 09 08 07 06 05

Through the Valleys is dedicated first and foremost to Jehovah Rapha, the God who heals. Praise his holy and healing name!

To my wonderful wife Julie, who encouraged me every step through this valley and whose weekly updates through e-mails kept God's people praying for me.

And to my children: Jordan, Jonah, and Jessica, who were there to make me laugh and inspired me to keep going.

To my parents, Ernest and Billie Sue, who agonized and prayed as they watched their only son fight for his life.

To the loving and supportive church I had the privilege to pastor for eight and one-half years, First Baptist Church, Odessa, Texas, who stood by their pastor in a critical time.

To my executive assistant, Glenda Daniell, for her help in correcting all my mistakes in this manuscript.

And finally, to all the saints around the world who prayed for my healing and recovery.

CONTENTS

Introduction

VICTORY COMES THROUGH THE VALLEYS

"YOU HAVE A VERY FAST-GROWING CANCER somewhere in your body." Now there are some words that will get your attention! My physician's words sent me into a tailspin. Suddenly, for the first time in my life, I was driven into a valley, not knowing if I would live or die.

If you live long enough, sooner or later you will find yourself in a valley. Valleys come in a variety of forms. The valley of fear. The valley of depression. The valley of financial ruin. The valley of divorce. The valley of discouragement, and the list goes on. Valleys are common and should be anticipated throughout life.

What God wants us to realize is that victory comes through the valleys. Valley life can lead to victory life when biblical principles are applied. In my valley of cancer, God taught me that he honors the prayers of his saints and the promises of his Word. Over and over God said to me, *"Ernest, you can trust me. You can trust me."*

God says to every valley dweller, *"Trust me. Trust me. Trust me."* From one valley dweller to another, let me tell you that God is faithful. You *can* trust him. He wants to take that valley of yours and turn it into victory. He did it for Bible saints like King Hezekiah, Jonah, Job, and others, and he can do it for you.

Today's valley is tomorrow's victory. No wonder the apostle Paul could say in Philippians 4:4, "Rejoice in the Lord always. Again I will say, rejoice!" *Through the Valleys* is a guide for those valley times. Chapter by chapter you will discover how God turns valleys into victory.

Jesus said in Matthew 10:27, "Whatever I tell you in the dark, speak in the light; and what you hear in the ear, preach on the housetops." That is what this book is about. The truths I learned while in the dark I am now speaking in the light. And what I heard God say while I was in the valleys, I am now preaching on the housetops.

Ernest L. Easley

The Valley of
UNCERTAINTY

2 Kings 20:1–11

"I have heard your prayer, I have seen your tears;
surely I will heal you."

2 Kings 20:5b

"YOU HAVE A FAST-GROWING CANCER somewhere in your body."
With that statement, I was thrown into the valley of uncertainty.
I was uncertain if I would survive. What about my family? Will
my life insurance policy be sufficient to meet the needs of my wife
and children? And what about our three children? Will they be
able to get a college education now? Who will walk my daughter
down the aisle on her wedding day? Welcome to the valley of
uncertainty!

Perhaps you are in a valley today. Your mind is racing with questions of uncertainty. You are not sure which way to turn. You are in
good company. The Bible is full of people who experienced valleys,
and lots of them! People of faith like Noah, Moses, Abraham,
Hannah, Job, Paul, and Silas, to name a few. They all faced the
valley of uncertainty.

One man in the Bible who found himself in the valley of uncertainty was King Hezekiah. He was the King of Judah. He had settled in as king, and suddenly he found himself in the valley of uncertainty. His story is recorded in 2 Kings 20.

THE KING'S CONDITION

We are told in verse 1, "In those days Hezekiah was sick and near death." For fourteen years, Hezekiah had served the people of Judah as king. He was comfortable. He was coasting through his administration and suddenly, wham! He was "sick and near death."

Hezekiah was suddenly thrown into a valley of uncertainty. That is how valleys usually come—suddenly. One minute you are coasting, and the next minute you are crashing. One minute you are healthy, and the next minute you are fighting for your life. One minute you have money in your pocket, and the next minute you are filing for bankruptcy.

Now being king, Hezekiah had available to him the best physicians and medical care. Money was certainly no problem. He had unlimited funds. But King Hezekiah soon learned that there are some things money cannot buy.

Verse 1 continues, "And Isaiah the prophet, the son of Amoz, went to him and said to him, 'Thus says the LORD: "Set your house in order, for you shall die, and not live."'"

On October 4, 1998, I discovered a knot on my lymph node in my neck while shaving one Sunday morning. The next week after an examination by my general physician, he suggested that I take a week's worth of antibiotics and come back.

During that week I went through my usual activities, noticing my lymph node increasing, not decreasing in size. After another visit with my general physician, he suggested that I see an ear, nose, and throat specialist. So that very week I walked into a strange building to see a specialist I had never met, to hear him say, "Let's take five needle biopsies from that lymph node."

Three days later I heard those dreaded words, "You have a fast-growing cancer somewhere in your body." I wish I could tell you that I stood firm, no concerns, saying, "Praise the Lord," but I cannot. The truth is that I went into shock and passed out for a few moments. I was grateful that my wife was with me. After the physician laid me back in the chair, placing a wet cloth on my forehead, he slipped out of the room for a few minutes.

No words were spoken as we tried to deal with being tossed into the valley of uncertainty. There are moments in the valley that require silence. Silence before God. Silence before man. Silence to contemplate. Silence to comprehend. God says in Psalm 46:10, "Be still, and know that I am God."

On October 12, 1998, my wife sent this e-mail to friends and family:

> I don't have a good report. After a long weekend of waiting, the first results are back from a needle biopsy Ernest had done Friday. He has been diagnosed with squamous cell carcinoma. He has a golf ball-sized mass on the right side of his neck that has doubled in size since he first discovered it. This fast-growing malignant cancer, we learned today, is not the source. It has just shown up first in his neck gland.

Tomorrow morning they will do a CAT scan in hopes of revealing the cancer source. After that, they will put him to sleep and do a panendoscopy. This means they will go down his throat and look in his ears, nose, esophagus, etc., in search of the main source of the cancer. I am trying to grasp what God has up his sleeve here. Either he is going to use this as an awesome platform to perform a mighty miracle, or he will use this as a wonderful example of how people who walk with God go through a time of trial and suffering. Either way he gets the glory. We are preparing for however God chooses to use this circumstance in our life.

THE KING'S PETITION

We read in 2 Kings 20:2–3, "Then he turned his face toward the wall, and prayed to the LORD, saying, 'Remember now, O LORD, I pray, how I have walked before You in truth and with a loyal heart, and have done what was good in Your sight.' And Hezekiah wept bitterly."

Several years before finding myself in the valley of uncertainty, I had been asking God to maximize my life for him. I would pray, *"Lord, . . . however . . . , whenever . . . , wherever . . . , maximize my life for your glory."* You need to know that if you do not really want God to maximize your life, don't ask him to. When you ask God to maximize your life, you place yourself in a vulnerable position before God. It is saying to God, "Whatever it takes, pleasant or unpleasant, painless or painful, maximize my life."

After packing our car to leave for M. D. Anderson Cancer Center in Houston, Texas, I went to our backyard to get alone with God. What the garden of Gethsemane was to Jesus, my backyard became to me. Not knowing what tomorrow would hold, with my hands lifted to the heavens and tears running down my face, I prayed: *"Lord, I have asked you for years to maximize my life for you. And knowing that nothing can get to me without first going through you, I know that you have allowed this cancer in my throat for your glory and my good. So, thank you for this cancer. I praise you for it. I do not know if I will live or die, but I do know that I can trust you. I know that somehow you are going to maximize my life through this valley of uncertainty."*

Forty-four radiation treatments will take their toll on you. For six weeks, five days a week, the radiologist would lay me down on a table and then secure my head with a meshlike mask. The actual treatment lasted only about ten minutes. As they laid me on the table for the first time, I was not sure what to expect. My mind raced to the New Testament book of Acts chapter 16, which records Paul and Silas in a Philippian jail. Verse 25 says, "But at midnight Paul and Silas were praying and singing hymns to God, and the prisoners were listening to them." I figured if it was good enough for Paul and Silas, it was good enough for me!

So during those ten-minute treatments, I prayed. I thanked God for saving my soul. I thanked God for my family. I thanked God for the radiation machine. I thanked God for the radiologist. And along with my praying came praise. I praised God for his faithfulness to me. I praised him for his goodness. I praised him for his mercy. I prayed and praised my way through all forty-four radiation treatments.

Now the treatments were painless, but their aftereffects were not. During the next ten weeks, I went from 190 pounds to 144 pounds. In one five-day period, I lost 15 lbs. I was slowly dying of malnutrition.

As I entered the fifth week of treatment, I could no longer swallow because of the hundreds of ulcers on my tongue and throughout my mouth and throat due to the radiation. So the physicians surgically placed a feeding tube directly into my stomach where it remained for six months. The feeding tube gave me a fighting chance.

Treatment by treatment my taste buds were being destroyed. Treatment by treatment my saliva glands were being destroyed. The outside of my throat was an open wound. And like King Hezekiah, I prayed to God and wept bitterly.

The valley of uncertainty is not always that severe. Sometimes it is more severe. But regardless of the depth and width of the valley, all valleys provide the child of God the best opportunities to bring the most glory to God. When life is smooth sailing and the waters are calm you say, "Praise the Lord! God is good," the world looks at you and says, "Well, of course they are praising God. If I lived in their house, drove their cars, and had their money, I would be grateful too."

But when the valleys come and the storms arrive and then you look up to heaven through teary eyes and say, "Praise the Lord! God is good!" the world will look on and say, "There must be something to Jesus after all. There must be something to knowing Christ after all."

The deeper the valley, the greater amount of glory and praise God gets. So if you find yourself in the valley of uncertainty, stop pouting and start praising. You will never have a greater opportunity to bring glory and praise to God than what you have today. The psalmist declares in Psalm 30:5, "Weeping may endure for a night, but joy comes in the morning."

THE KING'S EXTENSION

We read in 2 Kings 20:5–6, "Return and tell Hezekiah the leader of My people, 'Thus says the LORD, the God of David your father: "I have heard your prayer, I have seen your tears; surely I will heal you. On the third day you shall go up to the house of the LORD. And I will add to your days fifteen years. I will deliver you and this city from the hand of the king of Assyria; and I will defend this city for My own sake, and for the sake of My servant David."'"

If God came to you on your deathbed and said, "I have heard your prayers, I have seen your tears; surely I will heal you. I will add to your days fifteen years," how would you use them? Would you do anything differently? Would you love your spouse differently? Would you begin attending your children's sporting events rather than working late? What about your prayer life? Would it change? Would worship become a priority? How would you use them? Perhaps, more importantly, what about today? What about tomorrow?

Every day is a gift from God! "For what is your life? It is even a vapor that appears for a little time and then vanishes away" (James 4:14). Solomon gives us a wake-up call in Ecclesiastes 9:10, "Whatever your hand finds to do, do it with your might; for there is no work or device or knowledge or wisdom in the grave where you are going."

Don't assume that you have tomorrow. Don't put off something that needs to be done today, whether it is getting right with God; getting right with your spouse, your children, or your parents; or sharing the love of Jesus with a friend. Serve him every day! Share him every day! Show him how much you love him!

What are you doing with today's gift? Yes, today's gift may find you in a valley. What about Romans 8:28 where Paul says, "And we know that all things work together for good to those who love God, to those who are the called according to His purpose"? Does Romans 8:28 apply when you are in the valley of uncertainty? Absolutely yes! Ask Hezekiah.

During his valley of uncertainty, God deepened a passion for praise into his heart. Isaiah 38:9 says, "This is the writing of Hezekiah king of Judah, when he had been sick and had recovered from his sickness." After he expressed his struggle through his sickness, Hezekiah says in verse 19, "The living, the living man, he shall praise You, as I do this day."

Will you offer God praise today? Will you praise him through the valley? God honors the praise of his people, especially praise that comes from the valley. If you don't believe me, ask Paul and Silas. Back in Acts 16, after their praise service, verse 26 tells us that "suddenly there was a great earthquake, so that the foundations of the prison were shaken; and immediately all the doors were opened and everyone's chains were loosed."

That is what praise does: it sets prisoners free. Free of uncertainty. Free of fear. Free of the future. Praise honors God and God honors praise. You say, "But I don't feel like praising God." That is all the more reason to do it! If you wait until you feel like praising

God, you probably will never get around to it. But by praising God, you will then begin to feel like it.

King Hezekiah learned a timeless truth while in the valley of uncertainty: nothing can take you from here until God's plan and purpose are complete, and nothing can keep you here after God's plan and purpose are complete.

Every day is a gift from God, even those days that you find yourself in the valley of uncertainty. Praise your way through the valley, and experience the freedom found in Jesus.

The Valley of
FEAR

Isaiah 43:1–3

But now, thus says the LORD,
  who created you, O Jacob,
And He who formed you, O Israel:
"Fear not, for I have redeemed you;
I have called you by your name;
You are Mine."

Isaiah 43:1

WE ALL FACE FEARS. It begins in childhood and concludes in the grave. They are unavoidable. If you live long enough, sooner or later you will find yourself in the valley of fear. Not the helpful fears that keep you alive, but the hurtful fears that shorten your life.

I am talking about the kind of fear that drives you to your knees. The kind of fear that puts you into panic palace. And do not think being a child of God somehow exempts you. That's why God says again and again, "Fear not." Most of us are like the man who said, "I do not have any problems with eternal life and salvation and all of that; it is the next twenty-four hours that I'm worried about."

"I am going to give you forty-four radiation treatments in an attempt to save your life." As I heard those words from the lips of my oncologist, for the first time in my life, I experienced fear on a different level. I had experienced fear before but nothing like this fear. This fear drove me into temporary shock. Frankly, I wish I could tell you that when I was told I had a fast-growing cancer, I stood to my feet, raised my hands to the heavens, and shouted, "Praise the Lord!" But I did not.

As those words pierced my soul, I literally went into shock. The physician's lips were moving, but I could no longer hear the words. It was as though somebody muted the television set. I was numb. I was fear struck. As I was laid back with a wet rag on my forehead, there were no thoughts running through my mind. Totally blank. That is what shock will do to you. Welcome to the valley of fear.

After I preached one Sunday morning on valleys, a man walked up to me and said, "Pastor, have you ever noticed that all of the growth takes place in valleys? You never see anything growing on top of a high mountain, only in the valleys." And he was right! God knows that we need both mountaintop experiences and valleys to move us along in our faith. Yes, the mountaintop experiences are good, but the valleys are where we grow. The valleys deepen our roots of faith. The valleys drive us to God. Hosea 6:1 says, "Come, and let us return to the LORD; for He has torn, but He will heal us; He has stricken, but He will bind us up." God heals what he tears and binds what he strikes. Hosea reminds us that without experiencing his tearing, we would never experience his healing. Without experiencing his strike, we would never experience his binding.

The valleys develop our walk with God. No wonder Paul said in Philippians 4:4, "Rejoice in the Lord always. Again I will say, rejoice."

The gospel songwriter Andrae Crouch put it this way:

I thank God for the mountains

And I thank Him for the valleys

I thank Him for the storms He brought me through

For if I'd never had a problem

I wouldn't know that He could solve them

I'd never know what faith in God could do.

Even in the valley of fear? Even in the valley of fear! Is it possible? It *is* possible. When I reached the point of "thanking God for the valley" of fear, I then sensed his presence and peace. I did not want the valley of fear, but sometimes we need things we do not want. When I was a boy my parents said, "Ernest, you need a spanking." I did not want a spanking, but I needed one.

Sometimes we need things we do not want. At other times we want things we do not need. As a young boy, I wanted a Honda 70! I dreamed of riding it. But my parents knew that I did not need one. (They got smarter the older I got.)

Sometimes we need things we do not want, while at other times we want things we do not need. You may not want the valley of fear, but there are some things you will never learn without it. God wants to use that valley to drive you into a more intimate fellowship with him, to develop your walk and to deepen your faith. He wants to use the valley of fear to mold you into a person of faith. And as you walk through the valley of fear, you discover just how much you trust God.

In Isaiah 43, the children of Israel were in the valley of fear. Listen to what God says to his children in verse 1: "But now, thus says the LORD, who created you, O Jacob, and He who formed you, O Israel: 'Fear not, for I have redeemed you; I have called you by your name; *You are Mine.*'"

Do you hear that? The God that created and formed and redeemed you says, *"You are Mine."* Valley or no valley. Mountaintop or no mountaintop. Regardless of your circumstances. You are his! Nothing can change that, not even the valley of fear. What comfort! What peace!

That is what Paul was talking about in Romans 8:37–39 when he wrote, "Yet in all these things we are more than conquerors through Him who loved us. For I am persuaded that neither death nor life, nor angels nor principalities nor powers, nor things present nor things to come, nor height nor depth, nor any other created thing, shall be able to separate us from the love of God which is in Christ Jesus our Lord."

Would you stop for a moment, put this book down, and acknowledge God's presence today? Thank him for promising never to "leave you nor forsake you" (Heb. 13:5). Thank him that as you "walk through the valley of shadow of death, I will fear no evil; for You are with me; Your rod and Your staff, they comfort me" (Ps. 23:4).

"Lord, thank you for your unchanging word. Though in this valley I feel alone, I know that you are with me for you have promised me. Use this valley to teach me what I need to know. Help me keep my eyes on you as together we go through this valley. Give me that peace that surpasses all understanding through your presence. In Jesus' name I pray, Amen."

So what did God teach the children of Israel while in the valley of fear? More importantly, what value is there in the valley of fear?

Fears No Longer Need to Dominate You

"Fear not, for I have redeemed you" (Isa. 43:1). What a Savior! What a promise! As God sees you today in the valley of fear, he says, "You are mine. And because you are mine, unhealthy, unholy fear no longer has to dominate your life."

It is wonderful to belong to him and be known by him—especially when you are in the valley of fear. Especially when you are not sure what is coming next. What peace to hear God say again as he said to Isaiah, "For I, the LORD your God, will hold your right hand, saying to you, 'Fear not, I will help you'" (Isa. 41:13).

If you think that somehow you are holding on to God, I've got news for you. You are not holding on to him, but he is holding on to you. "For I, the LORD your God, will hold your right hand, saying to you, 'Fear not, I will help you.'"

To help keep our friends informed, my wife would send weekly e-mails. This helped keep rumors down and accurate information flowing so that people would know how to pray. On December 10, 1998, she wrote:

This past week has introduced many changes to his
physical and emotional condition. In the last six days, he
has lost fifteen pounds, *more* pounds. Convinced that he was
unable to eat and maintain his body weight, he agreed to
have a gastrostomy feeding tube inserted into his abdomen.
Dehydration was fast approaching. The sores in his mouth

get worse every day. Open ulcers hurt if anything touches them. The discomfort from the feeding tube is much less than the awful pain he has had trying to eat and drink.

Pray that it works like it's supposed to. It is very frustrating.

Early on during my illness and struggle with fear, I discovered Psalm 34:4, "I sought the LORD, and he heard me, and delivered me from all my fears," and Psalm 118:5–6, "I called on the LORD in distress; the LORD answered me and set me in a broad place. The LORD is on my side; I will not fear. What can man do to me?" Our problem is that we fear man so much because we fear God so little. But when we begin to have a healthy, respectful fear of God, our fear of man dissolves, not to mention our fear of the future.

Look again at Isaiah 43:1, "Fear not, for I have redeemed you; I have called you by your name, you are Mine." Do you see it? God says that you do not have to fear, regardless of the valley, regardless of the test reports, regardless of the situation, and here is why: "For I have redeemed you; . . . you are Mine."

Do you see the word *redeemed?* It means to release something, to deliver somebody, to buy something back. When God says, "I have redeemed you," he is saying that through the blood of Jesus Christ on a cross two thousand years ago, he purchased you, he bought you in order to release you from the bondage and burden of sin (including valleys).

When Jesus steps into your life, from that moment on, you belong to him. You are his purchased possession. Let me tell you something about fear: fear of the future is a waste of the present. That is, if you belong to him.

By the way, do you know what the opposite of fear is? It is trust. Valleys are times of trusting, not fearing. "The fear of man brings a snare, but whoever trusts in the LORD shall be safe" (Prov. 29:25). Fear and trust are extremes. They are opposites. You cannot be fearing while you are trusting, and you cannot be trusting when you are fearing. When fear moves in, trust moves out. When trust moves in, fear moves out.

Fear says to God, "I am not sure I can trust you with this situation. I am not sure you will come through. This valley may be too difficult for you to handle." It is when you are in a valley, trusting rather than fearing, that you discover "with God nothing will be impossible" (Luke 1:37).

FLOODS NO LONGER NEED TO DEVASTATE YOU

"When you pass through the waters, I will be with you; and through the rivers, they shall not overflow you" (Isa. 43:2).

Notice that he did not say, "*If* you pass through the waters." He said, "*When* you pass through the waters." Just put it down, you will experience times of flooding. I have had people say to me, "Pastor, I thought when I got saved that I would be free of struggles and storms." I do not know where they got that. Certainly not from the Word of God. Jesus said in John 16:33, "In the world you will have tribulation; but be of good cheer, I have overcome the world." We are told in Job 14:1, "Man who is born of woman is of few days and full of trouble."

God promises us that whether our flooding is ankle-deep, knee-deep, or neck-deep, we can know that floods no longer have to devastate us, and here is why: the presence of God! "When you pass through the waters, I will be with you" (Isa. 43:2). There is something calming and comforting about the presence of God. In his presence there is peace. In his presence there is comfort. In his presence there is rest.

One of the greatest fears I had to deal with concerned what I call *facing the facts.* Yes, I knew I had cancer. Yes, I knew it was a fast-growing cancer. But I struggled facing the facts.

I had been given a book on cancer several years before getting cancer. I kept it in my personal library. It described the various kinds of cancer, advisable treatments, and the odds of surviving. I knew I had the book. I knew right where it was in my library. And yet I could not read it for fear of what was in it.

After several weeks I worked up the courage to get it. I will never forget the fear and anxiety as I took it into my hands. I started by checking in the back of the book to see if *squamous cell carcinoma* was included. Sure enough it was. There were two references to this cancer. What would I find? Would I find that my family and friends and physicians had been withholding information from me?

Before I turned to the pages describing my cancer, God brought to mind a story I had read years before. A man came up to his pastor and said, "Pastor, I have found a great Bible verse on fear." The pastor asked, "What is the verse?" The man said, "It is Psalm 56:3, 'Whenever I am afraid, I will trust in You.'" The pastor said, "I have a better verse than that! It is Isaiah 12:2, 'Behold, God is my salvation, I will trust and not be afraid.'"

I decided that day to trust in the Lord and not be afraid, rather than being afraid and then trusting in the Lord. All of sudden, God released me of the fear that gripped me, and with confidence I opened the book. Trusting God in the valley of fear brings peace and strength. Acknowledging his presence brings assurance and hope. Are you trusting God today? Are you acknowledging his presence?

Here is what God said to Moses in Exodus 33:14: "My Presence will go with you, and I will give you rest." Here is what Jesus said to his disciples in John 14:16, "And I will pray the Father, and He will give you another [of the same kind] Helper [paraclete], that He may abide with you forever [everlasting]." Again David tells us in Psalm 23:4, "I will fear no evil; for You are with me." And in Isaiah 43:5, "Fear not, for I am with you," and in Isaiah 41:10, "Fear not, for I am with you; be not dismayed, for I am your God. I will strengthen you, yes, I will help you, I will uphold you with My righteous right hand."

God says, "I will strengthen you. I will help you. I will uphold you." Now let me ask you a question: How many different ways and times does God have to tell you something before you can trust him enough to release your unhealthy fear? You do not have to face any valley alone when you are his, regardless of how deep the water gets. Regardless of how strong the current gets. Fears no longer have to dominate you, and the floods no longer have to devastate you because of the presence of God!

Fires No Longer Need to Destroy You

"When you walk through the fire, you shall not be burned, nor shall the flame scorch you" (Isa. 43:2). Again, notice that he does not say, "*If* you walk through the fire," but rather, "*When* you walk through the fire." Just as floods will come, so will fires. There's no escaping the fire, but you can endure the fire. That is what God says here. "When you walk through the fire, you shall not be burned, nor shall the flame scorch you."

Do you remember the three Hebrew children? God did not take them out of the fire. Rather he took them by the hand and led them through the fire. He never left them or forsook them, and he will never leave you or forsake you. God has promised us, "I will never leave you nor forsake you" (Heb. 13:5).

Those three Hebrew children said to King Nebuchadnezzar in Daniel 3:17, "Our God whom we serve is able to deliver us from the burning fiery furnace, and He will deliver us from your hand, O king." King Nebuchadnezzar said, "We'll see about that."

He then tossed them into the flames and afterwards looked into the furnace and declared in verse 25, "Look! I see four men loose, walking in the midst of the fire; and they are not hurt, and the form of the fourth is like the Son of God."

Let me tell you something about that furnace: Jesus was there waiting for those three Hebrew children. He was already there. And just as he was there waiting for them to see them through it, he is waiting for you too. He was already there before you arrived. Before I lay down under that radiation machine for the first time, Jesus was waiting for me. When you belong to him, fears no longer have to dominate you. Fears no longer have to devastate you. And fires no longer have to destroy you. And as you go through the valley of fear, remember this.

God Is Faithful to His People

The apostle Paul said in 2 Timothy 2:13, "If we are faithless, he remains faithful; He cannot deny Himself." Valley or mountaintop, you can count on God. He is faithful, so be grateful. Because he is steady, you can be safe. He is faithful to you even when you are not faithful to him.

I can tell you that God has been faithful to me every step of the way, and he will be faithful to you. Next, God is faithful to his promises. The Bible says in 1 Kings 8:56, "Blessed be the LORD, who has given rest to His people Israel, according to all that He promised. There has not failed one word of all His good promise, which He promised through His servant Moses."

The apostle Paul declares in 2 Corinthians 1:20, "For all the promises of God in Him [Jesus] are Yes, and in Him Amen, to the glory of God through us." When you come across a promise from God, you can say, "Yes, Amen!"

God is faithful to our praise. Just as with Paul and Silas, the chains of bondage and burdens fall off as we give God praise. Stop pouting and start praising, for God is faithful to our praise!

When it comes to the valley of fear, there are two choices: when you fear, trust him, or trust him and not fear! When I found myself in the valley of fear, I tried both! My first response was fear followed by trust. Then when the trust began, the fear faded! Fear fades in the presence of Jesus.

"Behold, God is my salvation, I will trust and not be afraid; for . . . the LORD, is my strength and song; He also has become my salvation" (Isa. 12:2).

The Valley of
DETOURS

Genesis 37–50

"But as for you, you meant evil against me; but God meant it
for good . . . as it is this day, to save many people alive."

Genesis 50:20

HAVE YOU EVER TAKEN A DETOUR? You knew where you were going
and how you were going to get there, and you were on your way, and
then suddenly, wham! Detour! Perhaps a bridge was out, or a road
was closed for construction. Suddenly, rather than being on the main
road, you found yourself on a detour.

Nothing looked or sounded familiar to you. You did not plan
for it. You did not anticipate it. You did not see it coming. And yet
you found yourself detouring off the main road. If you live long
enough, sooner or later you will find yourself on a detour. And
oftentimes life's detours take you straight into a valley. Is that always
a bad thing? Not if you are a child of God, and here's why: victory
comes through the valleys.

My deepest valley, so far, came at age forty. I had life by the tail.
I was in my sixth year as the pastor of a growing, soul-winning,

mission-minded church. My beautiful wife and I had three healthy children. Our oldest child had just moved off to begin his college career. Our other two children were involved in church and school activities. We were making a difference for God! And out of nowhere came a detour. Well, not really out of nowhere, for nothing can get to us without first coming through God. But it sure looked like a detour at the moment, and so will yours.

Why does God place detours in our lives? And why do his detours often take us into valleys of uncertainty and fear? I will tell you why: to fulfill his plan for our lives. God is constantly working behind the scenes of our lives for his glory and our good! What he desires from us is trust!

We read in Isaiah 26:3–4, "You will keep him in perfect peace, whose mind is stayed on You, because he trusts in You. Trust in the LORD forever, for in . . . the LORD, is everlasting strength." The valley of detours will certainly reveal who trusts God and who does not. Sometimes we think we trust God, and we say we trust God. We stand up in worship singing, "Trust and obey, for there's no other way to be happy in Jesus, but to trust and obey," but do we really trust him? Do you know where you discover your trust level of God? In the valleys. In the testing times.

There was a young man who lived a long time ago who found himself in the valley of detours. His name was Joseph. When he was a teenager, God gave him a dream that one day his older brothers would bow before him. As you can imagine, when his older brothers heard about his dream, they refused to sit back and let it happen.

In fact, you will read in Genesis 37 that those sorry brothers decided to kill their youngest brother out of jealousy. We read in verse 18 that they "conspired against him to kill him." They then decided to seize him, strip him, and sell him, and that is exactly what they did. And young Joseph ended up in Egypt as a slave.

I would call that a detour that led to a valley, wouldn't you? And just when he thought it could not get any worse, it did. His detour landed him in the house of Pharaoh. We read in chapter 39 that while there, he was seduced by the beautiful wife of Potiphar, the captain of the guard.

I can imagine Joseph sitting underneath the stars that night, confused and contemplating, looking up into the heavens saying, "Lord, what did I do to deserve this? I have lived for you. I have honored you. And here I am on this unexpected detour. Why me? Why now? What do I do now?"

Sometimes when we see somebody in a valley, our tendency is to wonder what they did wrong. We think, *They must be living in rebellion against God to have experienced that.* Joseph wasn't rebelling against God. In fact, Joseph was in the middle of God's will, and he experienced the valley of detours. It wasn't that he did anything wrong; in fact, he did everything right. And yet God had a plan and purpose that required a detour in Joseph's life.

It could be that living for God has led you into a detour! That is why Paul said in Philippians 4:4, "Rejoice in the Lord always. Again I will say, rejoice!" Yes, even in the valley of detours.

How did Joseph turn his valley of detours into victory? And perhaps more importantly, how do we?

Count on the Promises of God

Rather than sinking on the premises, try standing on the promises. That is what Joseph did when he found himself in the valley of detours. God spoke to Joseph through two separate dreams that his brothers would one day bow before him. And when he found himself on a detour, not knowing which way to turn next, he counted on the promises of God.

Joseph must have thought that his detour would never end. He must have thought that he would never get back on the main road. But through the struggle and pain, he believed God's Word. He did not know how or when this detour would end, but somewhere along the way, God's Word would come to pass.

And look where his obedience to God landed him! It is found in Genesis 39:20, "Then Joseph's master took him and put him into the prison, a place where the king's prisoners were confined. And he was there in the prison."

He went from the pit to the palace to the prison. Now you talk about detours. I am sure his head was spinning. And yet Joseph knew that regardless of what happened, God would keep his word! Rather than dwelling on his problems, he was counting on God's promises. The result? He experienced *victory through the valley.*

It is not always easy to count on God's promises when you find yourself on a detour. For me it was helpful to have the support of a Christian wife, children, parents, friends, and church. Without their prayers and support, I am not sure I would have survived. As my radiation treatments began, my parents sent me a plaque with a passage of Scripture on it that they claimed for me throughout my illness. It was Jeremiah 29:11, "For I know the thoughts that I think toward you, says the LORD, thoughts of peace and not of evil, to give you a future and a hope."

My mother has been a prayer warrior for years. She had experienced over the years what James said in James 5:16, "Confess your trespasses to one another, and pray for one another, that you may be healed. The effective, fervent prayer of a righteous man [or woman] avails [accomplishes] much." And now with her preacher-son fighting for his life in a cancer center in Houston, Texas, on her knees before God, she begged God to heal me. She claimed Jeremiah 29:11, "To give you a future and a hope."

As I struggled to put one foot in front of the other on my way to radiation treatments, I wondered if it was worth the effort. Due to the radiation damage and large amounts of medication, for a couple of months I was sleeping up to twenty hours a day. When I woke up for either a feeding or a treatment, I wondered if I was going to live or die. After a four-week battle with nausea due to the large amounts of pain medicine I was taking, I wondered how much more I could take. And then I would glance over to that little plaque: "For I know the thoughts that I think toward you, says the LORD, thoughts of peace and not of evil, to give you a future and a hope" (Jer. 29:11).

I knew my family and friends were thinking about me. But to realize along the detour that God had thoughts regarding *me* was reassuring. He knew about my detour just as he knows about yours. And along the detour he has thoughts of peace and not of evil. He has given us a future and a hope. That was it for me. Detour or no detour, cancer or no cancer, nausea or no nausea, I was counting on the promises of God.

I was not sure if I was going to live or die. But either way I knew that through Jesus Christ I had a future and a hope.

COOPERATE WITH THE PLANS OF GOD

I have to hand it to Joseph: He cooperated with the plans of God. Joseph understood Romans 8:28, hundreds of years before the apostle Paul said, "We know that all things work together for good to those who love God, to those who are called according to His purpose."

One Sunday morning after I preached on this wonderful promise, a young man walked up to me and with great enthusiasm said, "Pastor, you quoted my life's verse in your message last Sunday." I thought to myself that he must be referring to Romans 8:28. I asked him, "What is your life's verse?" He said, "Job 14:1, 'Man who is born of woman is of few days and full of trouble.'"

Joseph could have claimed Job 14:1 as his life's verse too. I suppose we all could. But when Joseph found himself in the valley of detours, he not only counted on the promises of God; he also cooperated with the plans of God! And why not? He knew that God had a plan for his life, and wanting God's best, Joseph made a decision. And that decision was to cooperate with God. He decided to work with God rather than to work against him. No, the detour did not make any sense to Joseph, but Joseph knew that it all made sense to God!

Have you made that decision? Have you decided to work with God rather than to work against him? You say, "Ernest, how do I do that? How do I cooperate with God through this valley of detours?" How did Joseph cooperate? How does God want us cooperating with him when life no longer makes sense? *Joseph cooperated with God morally.* Remember this: You have an enemy with an agenda! Peter tells us this about this enemy in I Peter 5:8, "Be sober, be vigilant; because your adversary the devil walks about like a roaring lion, seeking whom he may devour." And just as God wants to bless you, Satan wants to blast you. While God is out to help you, the enemy is out to harm you! And one of the fastest ways the devil has of disrupting God's plans for your life is to tempt you morally. That is what he did with Joseph, and that is what he still does today.

Not once was Joseph tempted morally, but day after day. "Joseph was handsome in form and appearance. And it came to pass after these things that his master's wife cast longing eyes on Joseph, and she said, 'Lie with me.' But he refused" (Gen. 39:6–8). And then we read in verse 10, "So it was, as she spoke to Joseph day by day, that he did not heed her, to lie with her or to be with her."

Joseph made the decision to cooperate with God morally long before he was confronted by Potiphar's wife. By the way, that is the time to make that kind of decision. If you don't make that decision before being forced to make it, chances are great that you will make the wrong decision. God provides a way of escape with every temptation, even if it is just running. "But he left his garment in her hand, and fled and ran outside" (Gen. 39:12). Joseph remained in the proper position before God to receive his best by cooperating with him morally.

Joseph cooperated with God throughout adversity. It is not always easy to cooperate with God when life ceases to make sense. Granted, it is easier to cooperate with God when life makes sense, when you are on the main road, when you are not on a detour. But then suddenly, when you are confronted with a detour, cooperation sometimes goes out the window and is replaced with panic, fear, confusion, compromise, and even anger!

Through my detour valley, God taught me that walking with him in the light made it easier to walk with him in the dark. If you will walk with him when life makes sense, it is easier to walk with him when life doesn't make sense. I can tell you this: if you are not walking with God when life is smooth, your struggle will intensify when the lights go out.

I woke up Monday morning, October 12, 1998, walking with God and trusting him, not knowing I had a life-threatening cancer in my throat. I went to bed that same night walking with God and trusting him, knowing that I had cancer. Do not misunderstand me; I was devastated. I am just saying that I woke up that morning praising him, and I went to bed that night praising him. I have learned that you can praise the Lord and give him glory even through tears. In fact, praise lightens the load on the detour.

Can you imagine how Joseph felt when he was thrown into prison for *not* sleeping with Potiphar's wife? That was his reward for cooperating with God? Don't you know that Satan messed with his mind while he was in prison? He could have had the palace life, but now, because he had cooperated with God, he would have the prison life!

Then we read in Genesis 39:21, "But the LORD was with Joseph and showed him mercy, and He gave him favor in the sight of the keeper of the prison." And then in verse 23, "The keeper of the prison did not look into anything that was under Joseph's authority, because the LORD was with him; and whatever he did, the LORD made it prosper." In other words, when Joseph was up to something, the guard simply looked the other way! Don't tell me that God doesn't honor those who honor him!

Joseph cooperated with God in his prosperity. "Then Pharaoh said to Joseph, 'Inasmuch as God has shown you all this, there is no one as discerning and wise as you. You shall be over my house, and all my people shall be ruled according to your word; only in regard to the throne will I be greater than you.' And Pharaoh said to Joseph, 'See, I have set you over all the land of Egypt'" (Gen. 41:39–41).

Not only *morally* and in his *adversity*, but he included *prosperity* on the list. Joseph refused to allow anything to alter his allegiance to God, including prosperity. He had been given so much, and yet he remained faithful to God. Not one ounce of gold could cause him to turn his back on God. What a wonderful life principle! His prosperity did not alter his allegiance to God. The world could not provide enough things to cause Joseph to turn his back on God.

Joseph was determined to cooperate with the plans of God: *morally, throughout his adversity* and *along with his prosperity.* Have you made that determination? Have you ever said to God, "Regardless of what comes my way. Regardless how good things get. Regardless how bad things get. I am going with God." No wonder we read in Genesis 39:2, "The LORD was with Joseph, and he was a successful man."

Joseph took the valley of detours and turned it into victory! How did he do it? How do we do it? We must first count on the promises of God and then cooperate with the plan of God.

CLING TO THE PROVIDENCE OF GOD

What I was told at 4:00 p.m. on Monday, October 12, 1998, made no sense to me! One of life's biggest nightmares turned into reality when I was told that I had a fast-growing cancer somewhere in my body. There was nothing anybody could do about it except God!

One day while walking (more like shuffling) to a radiation treatment, my father, walking beside me, said, "Son, I wish it was me with the cancer! If there were some way I could take it from you, I would." But the reality of it was that he could not, regardless of how bad he wanted to! My children watched as their father was slowly losing weight and strength and perhaps dying, and they could do nothing to stop it. My wonderful and supportive wife, who never left my side, was comforting, but she too was unable to fix the cancer. It was God or nothing.

If you live long enough, a day will come when the only thing you have left to cling to is the providence of God. Just you with your problems and God and his providence. As one of God's children, I understood that nothing could get to me without first going through him. Did that make it easier through all of the suffering and sickness? Yes and no. Yes, I knew that somehow God would use this valley for his glory and my good. No, sickness is sickness and is never easy regardless of who is sick.

I have had people ask me, "Ernest, did it make any sense to you while you were fighting for your life?" No. But I knew it all made sense to God. And I knew that he would keep me in the valley of detours long enough for him to accomplish his will for his kingdom and my life!

Perhaps you are in the valley of detours today. You were just going through life serving God and suddenly, wham! The smooth road stopped and the uncertain detour began. From one valley dweller to another, let me tell you this: the detour will not last forever! There is a finish line to cross in the near future. You are closer today to that finish line than you were yesterday. Thank him for that. Praise him for that. You can know that God is at work while you are on this detour. The truth is that it is really no detour at all. Now to you it is a definite detour. But not to God. What a detour is to you is simply God working out his plan and purpose for your life.

At the time all Joseph could see was a prison. I am sure he had days when he felt that God had deserted him. After all, Joseph was a man like you and me. But he turned his valley of detours into victory and so can you!

Count on his promises! Cooperate with his plans! Cling to his providence! "The LORD was with Joseph, and he was a successful man" (Gen. 39:2).

The Valley of
SUFFERING

Job 1–2

And he said, "Naked I came
    from my mother's womb,
And naked shall I return there.
The LORD gave, and the LORD has taken away;
Blessed be the name of the LORD."

Job 1:21

"DR. EASLEY, THE FORTY-FOUR RADIATION TREATMENTS will be the toughest battle of your life." Those words came from a petite radiologist at M. D. Anderson Cancer Center who did not appear to have had a lot of suffering in her life. She was simply preparing me for the worst! After all, that was her job! Besides, she was not aware of my background.

She did not know that I was a Baylor University track letterman, who, through a lot of suffering and determination, became one of the top four hundred intermediate hurdlers in the Southwest Conference. I knew pain! I knew suffering! I knew physical battles! Boy, was I wrong! I was the one who had a lot to learn about

---

suffering. Cancer treatments brought a whole new definition of suffering and pain.

Welcome to the valley of suffering. Suffering is a common valley. To live is to suffer. You do not have to spend a lot of time at a cancer treatment center to know that suffering strikes at every age. God does allow it to "rain on the just and on the unjust" (Matt. 5:45). In other words, if you live long enough, whether you are a child of God or not, you will spend some time in the valley of suffering. Sometimes suffering is short and swift, but at other times it is long and slow. And the longer it drags on, the tougher it gets.

The valley of suffering is a common valley, but it can also be a confusing valley. You may feel abandoned by God. You may wonder if God really cares. You may feel abandoned by your friends. You may not know where to turn for help. But you can know that "the LORD, He is the One who goes before you. . . . He will not leave you nor forsake you; do not fear nor be dismayed" (Deut. 31:8).

What a thought! What a truth! That where you are today, God has already been! He was there waiting for your arrival. In fact, you cannot go where God has not already been, including the valley of suffering. And regardless of the severity of your suffering, you can know that no child of God suffers alone.

To learn more about the valley of suffering, an expert is needed. And if there was ever an expert in suffering, it was the man named Job. He not only models how to respond to suffering; he also illustrates how God honors those who honor him (I Sam. 2:30).

Job had it all. He had riches and respect. He had a reverence for God. He was a righteous man, and overnight he lost everything. Well, almost everything. As he entered into the valley of suffering, one thing he did not lose was his love for God. Here is a man whose deep roots of faith helped stabilize him when his suffering began.

As I began slowly recovering from my treatments, people asked me questions about my valley. One preacher asked, "How did you deal with the possibility of never preaching again?" That sounds like a question a preacher would ask, don't you think? I told him that preaching was not my biggest concern at the time, that I was more concerned about surviving.

Believe it or not, the local funeral director took me out to lunch and offered me a free funeral service, coaches included, if I would sign up for a pre-arranged funeral with his funeral home! (By the way, I refused his generous offer.)

One day, while I was still taking treatments, I received a letter from an elderly widow who wrote to tell me that she knew exactly what we were going through. It seems that her husband had the same type of cancer I had, but he died, and she hoped I would do better than he. I know she was trying to encourage me, but that was not what a man fighting for his life needed to read! After that, my wife began screening all e-mails and letters.

But the one question I have been asked most frequently is: "Did you ever ask God why? Why would God let this happen?" I honestly never asked God why. I asked, "Why not? Why not Ernest Easley?" After all, who was I to ask Almighty God, "Why?" I can tell you this regarding the valley of suffering: Victory comes through the valleys! If you do not believe me, ask Job.

THE ACCUSATIONS THAT JOB EXPERIENCED

To get a better understanding about the accusations Job experienced, you must first know of *his devotion to God.* We read in Job 1:1, "There was a man in the land of Uz, whose name was Job; and that man was blameless and upright, and one who feared God and shunned evil." You talk about stable! This man was sold out to God, "blameless and upright," meaning that he knew God intimately and served him! Add to it, he "feared God," which means that he knew the awesome power and majesty of God! No wonder he "shunned evil." No wonder he stayed away from things that displeased God!

Not only was he squeaky clean, but he also stayed the course of righteousness. He was a force for righteousness. Nobody questioned whether he loved God. He talked the walk and walked the talk. In fact, listen to God's six-fold description of Job, "Then the LORD said to Satan, 'Have you considered My servant Job, that there is none like him on the earth, a blameless and upright man, one who fears God and shuns evil?'" (1:8).

How would God describe your devotion to him today? How about *servant?* What about *none like him on the earth?* How about *blameless?* Or *upright?* Maybe *one who fears God and shuns evil?* Would you get one out of six? Two out of six? Three out of six? I'll tell you when these descriptions really begin to surface: in the valley of suffering! That is when you (and everybody around you) find out what is on the inside.

The next thing we discover is Job's dilemma before God. And that dilemma is recorded in verses 9–10, "So Satan answered the LORD and said, 'Does Job fear God for nothing? Have You not made a hedge around him, around his household, and around all that he has on every side? You have blessed the work of his hands, and his possessions have increased in the land.'"

In other words, Satan was saying to God, "The only reason Job is blameless and upright and fears you and shuns evil is because of what he has gotten out of it. With all he has, who wouldn't be good and godly?"

Listen to what Satan said next in verse 11, "But now, stretch out Your hand and touch all that he has, and he will surely curse You to Your face!" Then God responds in verse 12, "And the LORD said to Satan, 'Behold, all that he has is in your power; only do not lay a hand on his person.' Then Satan went out from the presence of the LORD."

Job's motives were being called into question. Satan accused him of being bought off by God. What about you? Why do you worship God? Why do you serve God? Is it because he is worthy of worship and service or because of what you think you can get from him? Would you worship him for nothing? Would you serve him for nothing?

There is nothing like the valley of suffering to reveal what is on the inside of a person. That is one reason God allows suffering. When I was in the deepest part of the valley of suffering, I realized that I did not worship or serve God because of his benefits but because of who he is.

Now don't misunderstand me; I appreciate and enjoy all of God's benefits. James tells us in James 1:17 that "every good gift and every perfect gift is from above, and comes down from the Father of lights." But that is not why I worship and serve him. I worship and serve him because of who he is. And I am not sure anybody can really know why they worship and serve God without a valley experience. You see it is true: Victory comes through the valleys!

Satan was on a mission to prove once and for all that people like Job were good for nothing. There was a mother who was exasperated with her five-year-old son who had been giving her fits most of the day. She said to him, "Son, would you please straighten up and be good?" He said, "I will if you give me five dollars." She looked at him and said, "Why can't you be good for nothing like your father?"

Well, maybe the nut doesn't fall far from the tree after all! Job, as you will discover, was indeed good for nothing, simply because of his love and devotion to God.

THE AFFLICTIONS THAT JOB ENDURED

Job suddenly found himself in the valley of suffering. There was financial affliction. We read in verses 14–16, "And a messenger came to Job and said, 'The oxen were plowing and the donkeys feeding beside them, when the Sabeans raided them and took them away—indeed they have killed the servants with the edge of the sword; and I alone have escaped to tell you!' While he was still speaking, another also came and said, 'The fire of God fell from heaven and burned up the sheep and the servants, and consumed them; and I alone have escaped to tell you.'"

First, he lost all of his oxen that were plowing, and his donkeys. Then he lost his servants and his sheep. And the valley kept getting wider and deeper. "While he was still speaking, another also came and said, 'The Chaldeans formed three bands, raided the camels and took them away, yes, and killed the servants with the edge of the sword; and I alone have escaped to tell you'" (v. 17).

Talk about having a bad day! He woke up that morning on top of the world! But before he went to bed that night, he was in the valley of suffering. The financial affliction began.

The valley of suffering often brings with it financial stresses—hospital bills, doctor bills, and lab bills, to mention a few. It does not take a lot of sickness to cause financial affliction. During a four-week period, the doctors could not find a medication that would stop my nausea. They tried and tried until finally they found something that worked. There were twenty-five little pills that cost three thousand dollars!

Fortunately, we had insurance. I was so sick I would have paid the full price. But I wondered what people did without medical insurance. In addition to good insurance, I pastored a loving and supportive church in West Texas. That church was a model when it came to caring for a sick pastor. And not only a sick pastor but also the pastor's family. They stood by us and made sure that no bill went unpaid.

Next, there was emotional affliction. We read in verses 18–19, "While [Job] was still speaking, another also came and said, 'Your sons and daughters were eating and drinking wine in their oldest brother's house, and suddenly a great wind came from across the wilderness and struck the four corners of the house, and it fell on the young men, and they are dead; and I alone have escaped to tell you.'"

About the time Job thought it couldn't get worse, it did. He not only experienced financial affliction; he also experienced emotional affliction! It was one thing to lose his fortune, but now his family?

One of the toughest things I had to do was to tell my family that I had cancer. When my wife and I came home from the doctor's office, still in shock ourselves, we somehow had to tell our three children (ages 18, 16, 14) the news. It was one of the worst nights of my life. First, to tell my children. Second, to notify my parents and my sister and her family.

I tried to tell my children but broke into tears before finishing. They went straight to their rooms where you could hear their wailing throughout the house. I then called my sister to break the news to her. I was in no shape to tell my parents that their only son had a fast-growing cancer, so my sister made that call. Our world, like Job's, came to a screeching halt.

What about Job's response to the financial and emotional affliction? Were Satan's accusations true or false? The answer is found in verse 20, "Then Job arose and tore his robe and shaved his head, and he fell to the ground and worshiped."

Look at it again. "He fell to the ground and worshiped." He turned his valley of suffering into a place of worship! "He fell to the ground [he got as low as he could get] and worshiped."

Would you call that a natural response to those circumstances? Of course not. His response was anything but natural; it was unnatural. Do you know what made that response possible? The same thing that makes it possible for you! He "was blameless and upright, and one who feared God and shunned evil" (v. 1).

There it is! That is the key! Whatever is on the inside will always spill out in the valleys. And listen to what spilled out of this man of God. "Naked I came from my mother's womb, and naked shall

I return there. The LORD gave, and the LORD has taken away; blessed be the name of the LORD" (vv. 21–22).

That is what spilled out: Faith rather than fear, praise rather than panic, worship rather than worry. Once you have your future secure, you can handle the present.

Yes, Job experienced financial affliction. And yes, he expressed emotional affliction. But Job also experienced physical affliction. After another conversation between God and Satan, and after Satan received permission again, we read, "Then Satan went out from the presence of the LORD, and struck Job with painful boils from the sole of his foot to the crown of his head" (2:7). Then we read, "My flesh is caked with worms and dust, my skin is cracked and breaks out afresh" (7:5). And, "My breath is offensive to my wife, and I am repulsive to the children of my own body" (19:17).

His physical affliction continues: "My bone clings to my skin and to my flesh, and I have escaped by the skin of my teeth" (19:20). And, "my bones are pierced in me at night, and my gnawing pains take no rest" (30:17). Then in verse 30, "My skin grows black and falls from me; my bones burn with fever." And yet we read, "In all this Job did not sin with his lips" (2:10).

Physical affliction is difficult to deal with regardless of its extent. I knew I was in trouble the fourth week into treatments. I had lost fifteen pounds in five days and could no longer swallow due to the ulcers in my mouth and down my throat. For a couple of weeks, my nutritionist had encouraged me to have a gastric feeding tube surgically implanted into my stomach in order to get the needed nutrients into my body. I had fought the idea from the start.

Looking back now, I suppose I equated that feeding tube with giving up and I was not giving up. (OK, I admit that I was not the best patient in the world.) Three nurses got me in a small room and jumped my case! I couldn't believe how they were talking to me. Didn't they know who I was? That was just it. They did know who I was: a cancer patient now dying of malnutrition because of stubbornness.

They won. The feeding tube was surgically placed directly into my stomach, relieving me from having to swallow my nourishment for six months. That feeding tube gave my body a fighting chance.

THE ASSURANCE THAT JOB ENJOYED

"Naked I came from my mother's womb, and naked shall I return there. The LORD gave, and the LORD has taken away; blessed be the name of the LORD" (1:21).

Where does that kind of assurance come from? After all the affliction he endured, how could he fall to the ground and worship God, praising his name and saying, "Blessed be the name of the LORD"? How could Job raise his hands in praise to God rather than shaking his fist at God?

The day before leaving for Houston, Texas, for treatments, I remember standing in my backyard alone with God. With tears streaming down my face, with hands raised to the heavens, I worshiped God! I praised him for his goodness. I thanked him for saving me. I thanked him for my family, my blessings, my church. I even thanked him for the cancer.

That's right. I thanked him for the cancer. Why would I do that? How could I do that? The same way Job could do it: he had put his trust in God. How do we know that? Because Job tells us, "Though He slay me, yet will I trust Him" (13:15).

Once you understand that God is sovereign, that he is King, and as sovereign God, nothing can get to you without first coming through him, you can then trust him! "Though He slay me, yet will I trust Him."

"You will keep him in perfect peace, whose mind is stayed on You, because he trusts in You. Trust in the LORD forever, for . . . the LORD, is everlasting strength" (Isa. 26:3–4).

Did Job understand all of his circumstances? Of course not. That was not the issue. The issue was whether he was going to trust God or not trust God. Job had learned to trust God because he knew God. And because he knew God, he loved God. Before you can trust, you must love. And before you can love, you must know.

Job knew God. Job loved God. Therefore, Job trusted God! And when life no longer made any sense, his trust was not shaken! Did God honor Job's trust? Look at Job 42:10: "And the LORD restored Job's losses when he prayed for his friends. Indeed the LORD gave Job twice as much as he had before."

During my sickness somebody gave me a copy of Dave Dravecky's book *Do Not Lose Heart*. In it he tells about a woman suffering from terminal cancer. Here is what she said to him in his own battle with cancer: *"The one thing that gets me through this as I lie here in my hospital bed is knowing every morning that, if God once more allows me to open my eyes, the first thing I'll see is a picture of Jesus hanging on my wall at the foot of my bed. When I see that picture of Jesus, somehow I get the strength to make it through another day."*

That is the way to get through the valley of suffering. By looking unto Jesus.

The Valley of STORMS

Matthew 14:22–33

But immediately Jesus spoke to them, saying,
"Be of good cheer! It is I; do not be afraid."

Matthew 14:27

I HOPE BY NOW YOU ARE BEGINNING to discover that victory comes through the valleys! As wonderful as mountaintops are, God allows us to experience the valleys for our good and his glory. The valleys are where we learn to trust and depend on God. That is where our walk with God gets closer and our faith deepens.

I can hear you say, "But isn't there another way? I mean, I want my walk to be closer to God and to have my faith grow deeper, but valleys? Can't God accomplish this another way?" That is probably what the disciples were thinking one night when they found themselves in the middle of a storm. But Jesus taught them some things in the storm that they would never have learned on the shore.

What kind of storm are you in today? The valley of storms can come in a variety of forms. Sometimes it is a spiritual storm. Peter tells us, "Be sober [calm], be vigilant [alert]; because your adversary

---

the devil walks about like a roaring lion, seeking whom he may devour. Resist him, steadfast in the faith, knowing that the same sufferings are experienced by your brotherhood in the world" (I Pet. 5:8–9).

At other times, it is a financial storm—the loss of a job, a financial reversal, and unexpected expenses. For many, it is a marital storm. Your spouse walks in and says, "I have had enough; I want out!" For you, it may be a physical storm. Sooner or later the storms will come and for good reason.

During my battle with cancer, I needed to know that what came to me had first to come through God! That is what Romans 8:28 means when Paul said, "And we know that all things work together for good to those who love God, to those who are the called according to His purpose." Do you see it? What comes to us must first come through him!

Knowing that before the cancer ever touched my throat, it first had to get through God gave me peace and hope. I realized that somehow God would use the cancer for my good and his glory. And not only for my good but also for the good of others.

The apostle Paul said in 2 Corinthians 1:3–4, "Blessed be the God and Father of our Lord Jesus Christ, the Father of mercies and God of all comfort, who comforts us in all our tribulation, that we may be able to comfort those who are in any trouble, with the comfort with which we ourselves are comforted by God." In other words, storms are not just for our good but also for the good of others! As we endure the storms, God comforts us. And then, in turn, we comfort others with the same comfort we received from God.

I cannot begin to tell you the dozens of people who were fighting throat cancer that God has brought into my life since October 12, 1998. I have been able to comfort and prepare them for the battle. I have been able to prepare and encourage them and give them hope. Sometimes God afflicts us on behalf of others. So don't waste your storm; invest it.

Rumors are inevitable, especially when you find yourself in a storm. One day a woman called our church office to speak to my secretary, Sandra Beard. She began telling Sandra how heartbroken she was regarding my struggle with cancer. She then asked Sandra if the "service" had been scheduled. Since we had multiple worship services, Sandra asked her which service she was referring to. She said, "Oh, the service for Dr. Easley. I just heard that he had passed away."

Though Sandra did not relay that message to me until months later, it greatly encouraged me. I told Sandra that I now knew there would be at least one person attending my funeral. To help cut down on rumors, my wife updated people through e-mails.

On October 12, 1998, six hours after I was diagnosed with squamous cell carcinoma, my wife Julie began her first of many mass e-mails by saying, "I don't have a good report" and concluded it by saying, "I am trying to grasp what God has up his sleeve here. Either he is going to use this (storm) as an awesome platform to perform a mighty miracle, or he'll use this as a wonderful example of how people who walk with God go through a time of trial and suffering. Either way, he gets the glory. We are preparing for however God chooses to use this circumstance in our life. We don't want to waste this experience." Don't waste your storm, invest it! Invest it in others!

Perhaps by now you are beginning to realize why it is not uncommon for Jesus' disciples to encounter the valley of storms. And though you may not be in a storm today, you can know that the storm clouds are gathering. There is no escaping it. "Man who is born of woman is of few days and full of trouble" (Job 14:1).

In Matthew 14, Jesus' disciples were still talking about Jesus feeding the five thousand with five loaves of bread and two fish. "Immediately Jesus made His disciples get into the boat and go before Him to the other side, while He sent the multitudes away. And when He had sent the multitudes away, He went up on the mountain by Himself to pray. And when evening came, He was alone there" (Matt. 14:22–23).

THE STORM THAT AROSE

As the unseen clouds were beginning to gather, we read of the Lord's instruction. "Jesus made His disciples get into the boat." The Greek word translated "made" is a forceful word. It means "to constrain them, to force them, to press them, to compel them" to get into the boat.

Now being the Lord of the seas, Jesus knew that a storm was brewing. You would think that because he loved them, he would instruct them to run for cover. But because he loved them, he "made His disciples get into the boat." In reality there were two storms brewing: one on the shore and one on the sea.

The storm on the shore is recorded in John's Gospel. "Therefore when Jesus perceived that they were about to come and take Him by force to make Him king, He departed again to a mountain by Himself alone" (John 6:15). No wonder they wanted to make Jesus king. Having fed five thousand men, besides women and children, with five loaves and two fish would ensure that nobody went hungry throughout the land. What they did not realize was that Jesus was already king, with or without their endorsement.

While a storm was brewing on the shore, a storm was also brewing on the sea. "But the boat was now in the middle of the sea, tossed by the waves, for the wind was contrary" (Matt. 14:24). It was time for the disciples to have their faith stretched, and Jesus used the storm to do it! Storms are like that, you know. They stretch your faith.

By obeying the word of God, the disciples headed straight into the storm. Were they led into that storm because of something they did wrong? No! In fact, they landed in the middle of that storm because of something they did right. They obeyed the word of God!

God uses storms in our lives for several reasons. He uses them for *correcting.* That is what happened to the prophet Jonah. Jonah rebelled, and God sent a storm to bring him back into fellowship with him.

God also uses storms for *perfecting.* That is what happened to young Joseph. God allowed Joseph to enter into a valley of storms to mature him and get him ready to be mightily used!

But God also uses storms for *instructing.* That is what we have in Matthew 14. God sent those men into the storm to teach them some things they would never learn while on the peaceful shore. For correcting. For perfecting. For instructing.

Sometimes we find ourselves in the valley of storms because, like Jonah, we have done something wrong. But at other times it is because we have done something right, like obeying the Word of God! Their obedience to Jesus landed them in a storm, a severe storm. We need to learn that God does not always lead us into a valley because we are disobedient. He sometimes leads us into a valley because of our obedience.

In Mark's account of this storm, we read about our Lord's observation. "And when He had sent them away, He departed to the mountain to pray. Now when evening came, the boat was in the middle of the sea; and He was alone on the land. Then He saw them straining at rowing, for the wind was against them" (Mark 6:46–48).

In every storm Jesus is watching. He sees you as you are rowing. He sees you as you are straining. "Then He saw them straining at rowing, for the wind was against them." The wind may have been against them but not Jesus. The apostle Paul wrote, "If God is for us, who can be against us?" (Rom. 8:31).

As you strain through the storm, keep in mind that Jesus is watching. He not only listens to you; he watches you. What does Jesus do as he watches you straining and struggling? Mark gives us the answer: "And when He had sent them away, He departed to the mountain to pray" (Mark 6:46).

First came his instruction. Then his observation. And finally, his intercession. As you go through the storm, he not only listens and watches, but he also prays.

Mark tells us that "He departed to the mountain to pray." Matthew tells us, "And when He had sent the multitudes away, He went up on the mountain by Himself to pray" (14:23). While they set out to sea, Jesus was back on shore praying for them.

Knowing that so many people around the world were praying for me gave me wonderful peace. On November 5, 1998, I received a letter from Bob Colin, one of God's great prayer warriors in Odessa, Texas. Here is a portion of that letter:

> We have just come back from Ridgecrest, North Carolina. On Wednesday night, the pastor of the week led a special prayer for you before preaching. The congregation consisted of people from eighteen states and countless churches, and many of them pledged to pray for you.
>
> In Asheville, we visited the Billy Graham Training Center called The Cove. There in the prayer room off the chapel, we offered a special prayer, and you were added to their daily prayer program.
>
> On the way home we stopped at First Baptist Church Albany, where you were prayed for at the men's prayer breakfast. On Monday and Tuesday I fasted and prayed. Do you get the idea that you are loved and are being prayed for?
>
> Lord, we join with the Easleys and thousands that are praying for healing in accordance with your will. Thank you for all the prayers you have answered on our behalf.

Jimmy Draper, president of LifeWay, concluded his letter to me, dated April 23, 1999, "Praying daily for you, Ernest!"

Claude Thomas, pastor of First Baptist Church in Euless, Texas, wrote on November 23, 1998, "Janice and I are praying for you as you go through this challenging time. Keep moving forward, and we will continue to join you in prayer."

Johnny Hunt, pastor of the First Baptist Church of Woodstock, Georgia, wrote on October 23, 1998, "Please know that I will continue to pray for you, and I will lead my church to pray for you." Then again on November 5, 1998, "I want you to know that not only did we pray for you in all three of our morning services with over five thousand present, but we also gathered all of our staff together on Tuesday morning and took you to the throne of God."

H. Edwin Young, pastor of Second Baptist Church in Houston, Texas, wrote on December 8, 1998, "Just a note to let you and your family know that you are in my prayers. I keep a personal prayer list on my desk, and you're right there."

Adrian Rogers, pastor of Bellevue Baptist Church in Cordova, Tennessee, wrote on October 19, 1998, "I have learned that you are going into the hospital for treatment. I want you to know that I love you and have prayed for you today."

It was wonderful to know that these men of God were praying for me, but it was not nearly as wonderful as knowing that Jesus was praying for me. And Jesus is praying for you.

"Therefore He is also able to save to the uttermost those who come to God through Him, since He always lives to make intercession for them" (Heb. 7:25). You can know that in every storm you encounter, Jesus is praying for you.

But what does he pray as he watches us in the storms of life? We are not told what he prayed that night while watching his disciples struggle. All we are told is that "He went up on the mountain by Himself to pray" (Matt. 14:23).

Perhaps he prays for us to trust him as we are rowing and straining. I can hear him pray for determination and deliverance for us in our struggles. Perhaps he prays for us to keep the faith and not to allow the storm to cause us to grow bitter but to grow bigger. I am not sure what all he prays, but I do know this: when the next storm blows across your life, you don't have to panic because Jesus is praying.

THE SAVIOR WHO ARRIVED

When the Savior arrived, his arrival was alarming. "Now in the fourth watch of the night Jesus went to them, walking on the sea. And when the disciples saw Him walking on the sea, they were troubled, saying, 'It is a ghost!' And they cried out for fear" (Matt. 14:25–26).

Jesus arrived during "the fourth watch of the night." That was from 3:00 a.m. to 6:00 a.m. He came to them in the storm, in the dark of the night. They could barely see their hands in front of their face. They certainly could not see the shoreline. They had no navigation machine to direct them. They did not know which way to go. And suddenly they saw Jesus walking on the water.

Isn't it good to know that Jesus comes to us in the storms of life? He is not just a fair-weather friend. Whether the sea of life is calm or contrary, whether the sun is shining or the waves are crashing all around us, Jesus is there!

God tells us, "I will never leave you nor forsake you" (Heb. 13:5). And yet, like those disciples, you may not always recognize him, but you can know that he is there. In the darkest hour Jesus came walking to them on the water, and in your darkest hour you can know that Jesus is there.

His arrival alarmed them. In fact, they thought that the phantom of the sea had arrived. That is what the word translated "ghost" means. This Greek word is where we get our English word *phantom*. His arrival was alarming.

It was also assuring. "But immediately Jesus spoke to them, saying, 'Be of good cheer! It is I; do not be afraid'" (Matt. 14:27). When he said that, they knew he was no phantom but the Lord Jesus! What they thought was going to be the worst thing that had ever happened to them turned out to be the best thing for them. The same is true for us.

I admit that when the doctor's report came back that I had cancer, I knew that October 12, 1998, was the worst day in my life. How could anything be worse? But now that the storm has passed, I realize that what I thought was the worst thing really turned out to be the best thing that could have happened.

Thousands of lives have received ministry through my storm. Even after two years since leaving First Baptist Church of Odessa, Texas, there are still cancer patients who call my former secretary inquiring about cancer treatment centers, oncologists, and asking questions about my treatments and recovery.

In fact, I was asked to tell my story at the 2001 Pastors' Conference at the Southern Baptist Convention. I stood that June afternoon at the Superdome and began telling what God had done, not knowing that the pastor search committee from Roswell Street Baptist Church in Marietta, Georgia, was in attendance. A few weeks later I was shocked to receive a call from Jerry Bonner, chairman of the search committee. He had heard me preach at the Southern Baptist Convention and wanted to know if I would be interested in visiting with him and his committee about becoming the next pastor of Roswell Street Baptist Church.

After it looked like I was going to live through this storm, I commented to my wife that I would never hear from another search committee as long as I lived. Now I was not complaining. I enjoyed pastoring in Odessa, Texas. But I could never imagine another church being interested in me because I would always be associated with cancer. My wife disagreed with me, which seldom has happened in our twenty-four years of marriage! She said, "Ernest Easley, you are wrong! What you have gone through and survived will cause other churches to want a pastor like you."

I truly thought that she was just trying to lift my spirits. But her insight was right again! The physical storm of cancer opened a door for me to pastor one of the great churches in the Southern Baptist Convention. What I thought originally was the worst thing that could have happened was really the best thing that could have happened.

What I thought was over my head was all along under his feet. Paul wrote, "And He put all things under His feet, and gave Him to be head over all things to the church" (Eph. 1:22). Wow! What a statement! What a truth! "And He [God the Father] put all things under His [Jesus Christ's] feet," and that includes every valley and every storm.

The Saints Who Were Astonished

Before that evening on the sea was passed, all of the saints in the boat would be astonished with the person of Jesus. "And Peter answered Him and said, 'Lord, if it is You, command me to come to

You on the water'" (Matt. 14:28). Isn't that just like Simon Peter? He always had something to say. Usually, the first screw that gets loose in a person's head is the one that controls the tongue!

Now don't be too hard on Peter. He was the only one in the boat who was willing to go to Jesus. He didn't care if he had to walk on the water or leap tall buildings. His desire was to be with Jesus.

Storms are like that, you know. Those who know Jesus want to be with Jesus, especially in the storms of life. Whether it was during my radiation treatments, or sitting through an hour-and-a-half feeding session, or learning how to swallow again, I wanted to be with Jesus. Many nights I enjoyed his company as we talked. Oftentimes I would wake up in the middle of the night talking to him. I would fall asleep talking to him and awaken again to pick up where we left off.

Now don't misunderstand me and think I was all alone. Nobody could have had a more faithful spouse. Nobody could have had a more faithful family. Nobody could have had a more faithful church and staff. But *nobody* understood or cared like Jesus. There is no better friend to have while in the storms of life than Jesus!

Next, we read about Peter's deed. "So He said, 'Come.' And when Peter had come down out of the boat, he walked on the water to go to Jesus" (Matt. 14:29). There it is! Peter walked on the water to come to Jesus. He stepped out of that boat, and he walked on the water to get to Jesus. Peter realized that in the storms of life, it is better to be out of the boat with Jesus than to be in the boat without him.

Next came Peter's doubt. "But when he saw that the wind was boisterous, he was afraid; and beginning to sink he cried out, saying, 'Lord save me'" (Matt. 14:30).

In just a flash Peter went from standing on the water to sinking in the water. And why? Because he took his eyes off Jesus and put his eyes on his circumstances. When Peter took his eyes off Jesus, he began to sink, and so do we.

As Julie drove us home from the doctor's office, having received my report, our attention was on the storm, and we began sinking. We sank spiritually. We sank emotionally. We were sinking fast, just like Simon Peter.

We are like that, aren't we? Adversity comes, the doctor's report comes, the accountant's report comes, and immediately the waves begin rising, and our attention heads straight to the storm. And then we begin to sink. And when it happens, you can know that you are in good company. The Bible is full of people who took their eyes off the Lord and placed them on their circumstances and began sinking.

Homes are sinking, churches are sinking, marriages are sinking, loves are sinking, countries are sinking, all for the same reason Peter began sinking: we have taken our eyes off Jesus! But there's hope. There is a way out for us, just as there was for Peter.

We read about Peter's deliverance. "And beginning to sink he cried out, saying, 'Lord, save me!' And immediately Jesus stretched out His hand and caught him, and said to him, 'O you of little faith, why did you doubt?'" (Matt. 14:30–31).

The good news is that regardless of how far you have sunk or how deep you have gone or how great the storm, when you pray,

"Lord, save me," you let loose the power of God. Waves and winds are no match for the power and presence of Jesus.

"Then those who were in the boat came and worshiped Him, saying, 'Truly You are the Son of God'" (Matt. 14:33). Regardless of how great your storm is, Jesus is greater.

The day after our life-shaking storm arrived, my wife Julie included in her second mass e-mailing, "It has been a long twenty-four hours. We have felt your prayers. It is unbelievable how God can calm the storm anytime we just trust him."

The Valley of

DISCOURAGEMENT

2 Kings 13:14–19

Yesterday God helped me,
Today He'll do the same.
How long will this continue?
Forever, praise His name.

AS MY FIFTH WEEK OF RADIATION came to a close, my wife began her
e-mail update with this greeting: "Hello from Cancerland!" After a
brief update regarding our children, she described my condition:

> His pain has gotten much more severe. His throat is
> covered with ulcers and blisters caused by the radiation,
> and he also has developed a bacterial infection in his
> mouth. Because these sores are all over his throat and the
> back of his tongue, it has become very difficult for him to
> talk. Try talking or eating without moving your tongue.

Talk about discouragement! I don't know anything that
will drive you into the valley of discouragement any quicker than
physical suffering.

Now I know what you are thinking: *But you are a Christian, a saint, a child of God! You are a pastor! Christians should never become discouraged, especially pastors.* I do not know where you got that, but it was not from the Bible. The Bible is full of God-fearing, Jesus-loving people who found themselves in the valley of discouragement!

Mighty Moses got discouraged. The prophet Jonah spent some time in the valley of discouragement. In fact, he became so discouraged that he wanted to die. And if you find yourself discouraged today, you are in good company. Do not think being a child of God somehow exempts you from the valley of discouragement. The devil works overtime to lead us into that valley to render us ineffective. If he can discourage us, he can defeat us.

That is what you find in the Old Testament book of 2 Kings. You will remember that God raised up a man named Elisha to continue the work of the prophet Elijah. Elisha had grown very sick. And if that was not bad enough, the old king had died, and his son, whose name was Joash, had just taken over the kingdom.

The young king was insecure and easily intimidated. He had no experience. He did not know whom he could trust. Now let me ask you a question: If you were the Syrians and you knew that Israel had an inexperienced and insecure new king, would you consider it a good time or a bad time to launch an attack?

That is what the Syrians thought too! They said, "The timing has never been better. Let's attack and take the kingdom." Word came to young King Joash that the Syrians were moving toward his borders with weapons in their hands and war in their hearts! Suddenly, the young king found himself in the valley of discouragement.

We too have an enemy who knows just when to attack. His attacks are strategically planned. He is out to derail and defeat you, and oftentimes he does it through the valley of discouragement. If he can discourage you, he can defeat you. And if he can defeat you, he can derail you from the tracks of holiness and usefulness.

Rather than being a victim of discouragement, how do you become a victor over discouragement? Perhaps it may be your health or wealth or some other life event which has driven you into the valley of discouragement. For you it may be your marriage. For me it was cancer! You may be so discouraged and disheartened today that you feel like walking away. People do it every day. Due to discouragement they walk away from a marriage, a job, or a church.

Is there a way through the valley of discouragement? The answer is a resounding yes! Just ask King Joash. Where do you begin in becoming a victor over discouragement rather than being a victim of discouragement?

Place Your Discouragement in the Hands of God

That is the place to start in defeating discouragement. Place your discouragement in the hands of God. That is what Joash did. "And Elisha said to him, 'Take a bow and some arrows.' So he took himself a bow and some arrows. Then he said to the king of Israel, 'Put your hand on the bow.' So he put his hand on it, and Elisha put his hands on the king's hands" (2 Kings 13:15–16).

Did you notice whose council the king sought? The prophet of God, that's who. Not the astrologers, not the wizards, not the prophets of Baal. He sought the council of a man of God! "Then

Joash the king of Israel came down to him [Elisha]" (v. 14). Do you see it? He stepped down off his high and mighty throne and headed straight to Elisha, a man of God, for council and wisdom!

Discouraged? Then let me ask you a question: Are you seeking godly council or worldly council? The direction you head for council speaks volumes about your view of God as well as your walk with God.

I was grateful for the godly council I received during my valley of discouragement. I was confused and not thinking clearly when I was told I had throat cancer. My mind raced with questions: *Where do I seek treatment? Which physicians can I trust? What will happen to my family? What will happen to the church I pastor?* As I placed my trust in God, he supplied an answer and direction for every concern, and often in spite of my ignorance!

My dear pastor friend from Austin, Texas, Ralph M. Smith, had nearly died several years prior to my cancer. I watched him literally fight for his life. If ever a man knew about discouragement and pastoring, I knew it was Ralph Smith. I received a letter from him dated October 19, 1998, seven days after I was told about my cancer. Now that is a friend! Never underestimate the power of the pen.

Dear Ernest,

I think of you every day. I pray you are better daily. Seems you are going to have a process before you whip this problem. Let me tell you what I did while in the hospital thirteen months and following:

First, I did nothing. That was all I could do. Second, I prayed. I have never prayed so much for my family. Third, I tried to encourage my wife and family. They were having a harder time than me, though in a different way. Fourth, I tried not to worry about the church. It was there before I came and is doing well since I left. Oh yes, you will not like all they will do, but so what! Fifth, I worked on my sense of humor. I learned to chuckle inside when they could not get the needle in the vein or when I wanted a nurse and she was nowhere around. "This too shall pass" became my motto. Sixth, maybe this was first, I got a layman in the church to be my wife's financial advisor. Seventh, I did not try to return calls, cards, or worry about commitments I had made for speaking engagements, weddings, etc. Someone else would need to take care of that. I quickly realized my main concern was getting my health back, everything else would have to be put on hold.

Know I love and appreciate you.

Your Friend,

Ralph

Discouragement is a time to seek godly council. Seek godly council. And not only their council but their prayers. "The effective, fervent prayer of a *righteous man* avails much" (James 5:16). You want "righteous" people, those in right standing with God, those who walk with God and love God, praying for you when you are in a valley. Why? Because their prayers accomplish much!

That is what King Joash did. He sought godly council and support. "Elisha had become sick with the illness of which he would die. Then Joash the king of Israel came down to him, and wept over his face . . . . And Elisha said to him, 'Take a bow and some arrows.'

So he took himself a bow and some arrows. Then he said to the king of Israel, 'Put your hand on the bow.' So he put his hand on it, and Elisha put his hands on the king's hands" (2 Kings 13:14–16).

After grabbing his bow and arrow, he brought them to the old prophet. Elisha put his hands on the hands of the young king and blessed his hands, his talents, his weapons, and his skill.

As Elisha laid his hands on the hands of the king, I can hear him praying, "Dear Lord, bless this young king. Give him courage! Give him wisdom! Give him victory over all his enemies! May his life and lips honor you!"

Just as the laying on of hands in the New Testament was associated with committing and consecrating a man to God, the laying on of Elisha's hands on the hands of King Joash was his way of placing him in the hands of God. That is the place to start when you are discouraged. Place your discouragement in the hands of God. Bring that discouragement and lay it before him and let his hands rest on your hands.

Our problem is that we are fighting God's battles. Do you remember what David said to Goliath just before that giant was defeated? "For the battle is the LORD's, and He will give you into our hands" (1 Sam. 17:47). Quit fighting his battles. No wonder you are defeated with discouragement. "Trust in the LORD with all your heart, and lean not on your own understanding; in all your ways acknowledge Him, and He shall direct your paths" (Prov. 3:5–6).

The apostle Paul tells us in 2 Corinthians 1:3, "Blessed be the God and Father of our Lord Jesus Christ, the Father of mercies and God of all comfort." When Paul described God the Father as the "God of all comfort," the Greek word that is translated "comfort" (*parakleseos*) means "encouragement." In other words, he is the God of all encouragement. God brings encouragement into our lives to off-set the devil's discouragement, as we bring our problems and pains to him, allowing his hands to rest on ours.

Let me ask you two questions: Is your discouragement bigger than the hands of God? Do you know what discouragement really is? It is forgetting God. King Joash took his focus off God and onto the army of the Syrians. And when he did that, he moved into the valley of discouragement. When Simon Peter took his eyes off Jesus and onto the troubled sea, discouragement set in and he sank.

It happens every time. Discouragement comes when you forget God. Have you forgotten God today? Has your focus been placed upon your enemies who are attacking? Is there victory through the valley of discouragement? Yes. And the first step is to place your discouragement in the hands of God.

REPLACE YOUR DISCOURAGEMENT WITH ACTION

Having placed his discouragement in the hands of God, we read next that Joash then replaced his discouragement with action. "And [Elisha] said, 'Open the east window'; and he opened it. Then Elisha said, 'Shoot'; and he shot" (2 Kings 13:17).

King Joash shot his way out of discouragement by taking the initiative. He moved from inactivity to activity. The worse thing you can do while in the valley of discouragement is to stay by yourself and do nothing! Discouraged? Take action! Get up! Get going! What good will that do? Well, to begin with, it will get you out of inactivity. That is what Elisha told Joash to do: Get up and move into action.

I suppose one of the great battles fought while in the valley of discouragement is against becoming lethargic, that "I don't feel like doing anything" feeling. That is what the valley of discouragement does. It moves you into lethargic living. Have you ever been there? Our tendency is to wait until we feel like doing something before we actually do something! Perhaps you have heard the expression, I will do it when I feel like doing it. Chances are great, then, that you will never do it.

A valuable life lesson I learned while in the valley of discouragement is that by acting something out, feelings will follow. First comes action and then come feelings. For instance, you say, "I don't read my Bible because I don't feel like doing it." I can guarantee then that the devil will see to it that you never feel like reading the Word of God! But if you begin reading it, feeling or no feeling, you will start feeling like it. First comes action and then come feelings. Feelings follow actions.

Or somebody says, "When I feel like cleaning my room, then I'll clean it." If so, your room will resemble a pig sty. Our struggle is that we want to get it on the inside first. *When I feel like it, then I'll start doing it.* When Joash opened that window and shot that arrow, it was his way of saying, "I'm going to face my enemy! I am going to do something. I am going to replace my discouragement with action." Enough of lethargic living. It is time to move into action.

Face Your Discouragement with Faith

As Joash shot that arrow, Elisha said, "The arrow of the LORD's deliverance and the arrow of the deliverance from Syria"

(2 Kings 13:17). Do you know what you need to shoot your discouragement? An arrow of faith! That is what Joash did. He shot his discouragement with an arrow of faith!

How do you face your discouragement with faith? How did Joash do it? Well, after receiving the word of God from Elisha, he obeyed it! That's right! He simply obeyed it. That is the key for turning valleys into victory.

Obedience. Valley or no valley. Mountaintop or no mountaintop and here is why: Bible faith is obeying the Word of God. When you do what God says, you exercise faith. "But without faith it is impossible to please Him" (Heb 11:6).

Joash exercised faith by obeying the word of God. And because he obeyed God's word, he received God's blessing. And with that blessing came God's power. And God's power enabled him to experience victory through the valley of discouragement.

Now let me ask you a simple question: Could Joash defeat the mighty Syrian army by shooting one little arrow into the air? Come on. One arrow? How silly to think he could defeat the Syrians by shooting one arrow out the eastern window. Do you think he really thought that somehow one arrow could give him victory? I think he did and here is why: Joash knew enough to know that obedience to the word of God would ultimately mean victory. You can never go wrong when you obey the word of God.

Joash obeyed the word of God, which took faith. And because he exercised his faith, God moved in. And when God moved in, he supplied the power for the victory. Every discouraged saint needs to learn what Joash learned: one + God = a majority.

You say, "But Ernest, my circumstances seem impossible." Wonderful! Now God can work a miracle, because with God nothing is impossible! I read years ago somewhere that problems are platforms for God to do a miracle. Had Bartimaeus not been born blind, Jesus would never have given him sight. Had the leper not had leprosy, Jesus would never have healed him. Had Lazarus not died, Jesus would never have raised him from the dead. Problems really are platforms for God to work a miracle. "I can do all things through Christ who strengthens me" (Phil. 4:13). "For with God nothing will be impossible" (Luke 1:37).

Erase Your Discouragement with Persistence

"Then he said, 'Take the arrows'; so he took them. And he said to the king of Israel, 'Strike the ground'; so he struck three times, and stopped. And the man of God was angry with him, and said, 'You should have struck five or six times; then you would have struck Syria till you had destroyed it! But now you will strike Syria only three times'" (2 Kings 13:18–19).

Do you know why Elisha was angry with the king? The same reason you get defeated by discouragement: he quit too soon. Discouraged people often quit too soon and miss out on God's best. I suppose one of the hardest things to do in life is to keep going when you feel like quitting.

My wife Julie included this update in her daily (sometimes weekly) e-mail on December 10, 1998, "This past week has introduced many changes to his physical and emotional condition. Between Tuesday, December 1, and Monday, December 7, he lost fifteen more pounds. Convinced that he was unable to eat and maintain his body weight, he agreed to have a feeding tube installed in his abdomen."

What she didn't tell is the battle I put up regarding that feeding tube. I had been told from the start that I would need one. Every week that passed I would be asked, "Are you ready for the feeding tube?" And every week they would get the same answer, "No, I'm fine."

I was not fine. I was stubborn and hardheaded. Finally, my nutritionist, radiologist, nursing assistant, and my wife put me in a small room. They sat me in a chair and gave me the third degree! They asked me why I was so stubborn. They asked me how much longer I thought I could live without a feeding tube. They asked me who I thought I was to ignore their recommendation. And looking back, I think their plan was to keep me in there until I finally screamed "uncle."

In my mind, giving up to have the feeding tube was like throwing in the towel. But looking at it now, agreeing to a feeding tube was agreeing to keep on fighting. What little fight I had left gave me the courage to press on, tube and all.

To you the discouraged, let me pass something along to you I learned in my valley of discouragement: hang in there until the circumstances change, and in the process, you will change. Somebody once said that "persistence is sticking to something that you are not stuck on." It is often the last key on the ring that opens the door. It is always too soon to quit. Stopping at third base adds no more to the score than striking out.

The Valley of
CONFUSION

Habakkuk 1–3

O LORD, how long shall I cry,
And You will not hear?
Even cry out to You, "Violence!"
And You will not save.

Habakkuk 1:2

OVER TWENTY-FIVE HUNDRED YEARS AGO, there was a prophet named Habakkuk, who looked around one day and saw his world falling apart and doubted if God cared about him. He was frustrated with God and no wonder. After all, his world was spinning out of control, and to make matters worse, it seemed to him that God didn't care.

Sooner or later life will take you into the valley of confusion. When life no longer makes any sense to you, you can know that you have arrived in the valley of confusion. You look around and ask, "Why are things the way they are? When will they change?" You will say, "It's not supposed to happen this way. This cannot be happening to me. Not me. Not now. Not ever!"

Those were some of my earliest thoughts after discovering that I had a fast-growing cancer in my throat. *This could not be happening. Not to me. Not now. Not ever!* When a crisis strikes, when unwelcomed or unprepared circumstances suddenly arrive, it is not uncommon to experience confusion.

Here is a valley the devil loves to see you in. Since he cannot destroy you as a child of God, he works overtime to defeat you. And when confusion comes, he steps in and begins playing with your mind. He will suggest that if God really cared, he would step in to help you or heal you.

When sickness or sorrow enters your world and you pray for healing or help and it doesn't seem that God is doing anything, you can quickly begin wondering if there is a God. And if there is a God, does he care? And if he cares, why doesn't he step in and stop all of this?

While spending time in the valley of confusion, I discovered that it is not easy to keep it all together when your world is falling apart. Not emotionally. Not spiritually. Not physically. During times of confusion, we need to do what Habakkuk's name suggests: to embrace Almighty God. Embrace his promises. Embrace his word. Embrace his will. Embrace him. Firmly cling to God regardless of what happens.

That is what the Hebrew name *Habakkuk* means, "to embrace, to cling to." When I was confused the most, I embraced the most. I decided early on that whether I lived or died, whether I was healed or not, I was clinging to God. I chose to embrace him through every treatment and every test. It is true: there is victory through the valleys.

That is what this Old Testament prophet named Habakkuk discovered. He took his confusion and frustration to God and found the answers to his deepest questions.

The Problems That Confused Him

Problems are oftentimes confusing. They sure were for Habakkuk, who looked around his world and began wondering where God was. Habakkuk begins with a complaint to God, "O LORD, how long shall I cry, and You will not hear? Even cry out to You, 'Violence!' and You will not save" (Hab. 1:2). As his world began to unravel, Habakkuk prayed and prayed, and yet heaven was silent!

Have you ever prayed and prayed and did not seem to get an answer? Perhaps your world is falling apart these days and you are praying persistently, and yet there does not seem to be an answer from God. You may feel like Habakkuk who asked God, "How long shall I cry, and You will not hear?" In the same verse he goes on to say, "Even cry out to You, 'Violence!'"

In the English it appears that Habakkuk uses the same word "cry" two separate times. But in the Hebrew they are two distinct words. When he asks, "How long shall I cry, and You will not hear?" the Hebrew word that is translated "cry" speaks of a cry or plea for help. When he says, "Even cry out to You, 'Violence!'" the Hebrew word that is translated "cry" speaks of shouting. He really lets God have it, as though God has grown hard of hearing!

In other words Habakkuk began with a plea and ended with a shout to God. His frustration and confusion had built up like steam in a teakettle, and the lid finally gave way to the pressure. It is frustrating when you are confused and heaven seems to be silent. Matthew Henry reminds us that "the God of Israel, the Savior, is sometimes a God that hides himself but never a God that is absent; sometimes in the dark, but never at a distance."

Habakkuk's complaint to God was largely due to his circumstances before God. He goes on to say, "Why do You show me iniquity, and cause me to see trouble? For plundering and violence are before me; there is strife, and contention arises" (Hab. 1:3). No wonder he was confused! God showed him the moral decay of his day. He said to God, "Why do You show me iniquity?"

Whose iniquity was God referring to? The people of God, that's who! Not the sin of the ungodly, but the godly! Habakkuk saw the so-called "believers" who had been blessed by God living like "unbelievers." They were disregarding the word of God in their everyday lives. Their lifestyles were bringing disgrace on God's grace! They were bringing shame to the name of God!

Sound familiar? It sounds to me like he was describing the twenty-first-century church! This prophet saw even more. Not only the moral decay of the people of God, he also saw their spiritual decline. Moral decay and spiritual decline. "For plundering and violence are before me; there is strife, and contention arises" (v. 3).

Listen again to what Habakkuk saw among the people of God: iniquity, trouble, plundering, violence, strife, contention. A far cry from Leviticus 11:44, "For I am the LORD your God. You shall therefore consecrate [set apart from the world and set apart unto God] yourselves, and you shall be holy; for I am holy."

A far cry from Exodus 11:7, "You may know that the LORD does make a difference between the Egyptians [*world*] and Israel [*people of God*]." There is something wrong when Christians live like, sound like, act like, and respond like their lost neighbors.

Habakkuk saw all of that and cried out, "God, where are you? How can you do nothing about all of this? How can you continue putting up with all of this?" He could not understand why God wasn't stepping in and doing something about the situation.

I have to admit that there were days when I wondered why God did not step in and do something about my cancer. Why wouldn't he touch me like he touched the leper who was instantly cured? I knew that he could do it. Why would he not do for me what he did for blind Bartimaeus who instantly received his sight? I'll tell you why: Because he was doing something in Ernest Easley that he didn't do in the leper and Bartimaeus. His plan for me was different from his plan for that leper and Bartimaeus. And I'll take that one step further: God is doing some things in you that he didn't do in me, and his plan for you is different from his plan for me.

What God wants to know is whether you trust him. And frankly, you really do not know if you trust God until you have to— that is, not until he's all you have left. It is easy to say, "Of course I trust God." It is another thing to be in the valley and trust God.

The psalmist declares, "Whenever I am afraid, I will trust in You. In God (I will praise His word), in God I have put my trust; I will not fear" (Ps. 56:3–4). How wonderful that when we are afraid, we can trust God. But as wonderful as that is, there is something even more wonderful. The prophet Isaiah declares in Isaiah 12:2, "I will trust and not be afraid; For YAH, the LORD, is my strength and song; He also has become my salvation." Do you hear the difference? Why be afraid and trust God when you can trust God and not be afraid?

Need more proof? God tells us in Isaiah 41:10, "Fear not, for I am with you; be not dismayed [confused], for I am your God. I will strengthen you, yes, I will help you, I will uphold you with My righteous right hand." What a God! He tells us that he will strengthen you, help you, and uphold you with his righteous right hand!

Habakkuk was confused due to the problems that he saw. First came his complaint to God. Second, we read about *his circumstances before God.* And then suddenly came the confirmation from God.

Just when he was about to give up, just when he thought God was not listening, God answered. God's silence does not mean God is not listening. You can know that God is listening through every valley. He heard you early this morning. He heard you when you asked him to heal your broken heart. He heard you cry out to him in your frustration. Because he loves, he listens.

Habakkuk discovered that though it seemed God was inactive, he was involved all the time! As I lay on the radiation table five days a week for over two months, at times it did not seem that God was involved. Day after day I cried out to him in my confusion for a miracle. I soon learned what Habakkuk learned, that God's involvement is not determined by his silence but by his sovereignty. He remains on the throne of the universe through your every valley.

What did God confirm to Habakkuk? He confirmed that he was not going to allow all the sin that Habakkuk saw go unpunished. Basically, God told him, "You think things are bad now? You haven't seen anything yet." For we read, "Look among the nations and watch—be utterly astounded! For I will work a work in your days which you would not believe, though it were told you. For indeed I am raising up the Chaldeans, a bitter and hasty nation which marches through the breadth of the earth, to possess dwelling places that are not theirs. They are terrible and dreadful" (vv. 5–7).

The Chaldeans were the Babylonians (modern-day Iraq). God said that he had raised up the ungodly, the impure, the unrighteous to judge Israel. In other words, he is going to judge the godly, and he's going to use the ungodly to do it. Habakkuk could not believe it. It did not make any sense. Of all the people in the world, the Chaldeans? So Habakkuk responded to God in verse 12, "Are You not from everlasting, O LORD my God, my Holy One? We shall not die. O LORD, You have appointed them for judgment; O Rock, You have marked them for correction."

Isn't that just like us? Especially in the valley of confusion when we tend to tell God how to do his job. And God said to him, "I told you that you wouldn't believe it." May I remind you today that God knows what he is doing. Your circumstances may have you confused today, but you can rest assured that God knows what he's doing. What he wants from you is trust, even in the valley of confusion.

THE PROMISES THAT COMFORTED HIM

God's answer is often not what we anticipate, but it is always what we need. In fact, while in the valley of confusion, Habakkuk learned not to live by presumptions but by promises—God's promises. After all, that is what trust is all about. And not just "standing on the promises" but "living by the promises." That is the only way to endure the valley of confusion, by both standing and living on the unchanging promises of God.

What promises did God use to comfort this confused prophet? The same promises that he uses to comfort us. For instance, the promise that God's Word is trustworthy. "Write the vision and make it plain on tablets, that he may run who reads it" (Hab. 2:2). Habakkuk did write it down on tablets, and it was later divided into three chapters. Today we know it as the book of Habakkuk.

Why would God want him to write this information down on tablets? The answer is partially found in verse 3, "For the vision is yet for an appointed time; but at the end it will speak, and it will not lie." God instructed Habakkuk to record this vision because his Word is absolutely trustworthy. Even in the valley of confusion? Even in the valley of confusion. Even when your life is coming unraveled? Even when your life is coming unraveled. You can trust the Word of God in every circumstance. In every valley, in every crisis, in every storm, in every reversal. God's Word is absolutely trustworthy.

Near the end of my treatments, I was in such pain that my oncologist decided to prescribe a heavy dosage of Lortab for me. I had long passed Demerol and Percocet for pain. The radiation had produced hundreds of ulcers in my mouth and down my throat. My throat was so damaged I could no longer drink water. The feeding tube was used not only for my meals and medication but also for all liquids.

When your body is running on Lortab, it not only reduces the pain, but it also reduces your comprehension. I remember one afternoon, picking up my Bible, reading a single verse of Scripture, and before finishing it I could not remember what it said at the beginning of the passage. I thought, *Ernest, you are not concentrating! Catch your breath and read the next verse.* I tried again only to find the same result. I suddenly realized that I could not read one sentence, one passage, or one verse and remember what I had read, regardless of how much I tried.

I sat there in a chair thinking, *How am I going to get through this without feeding on God's Word? I cannot even comprehend a four-word passage of Scripture?* I quietly closed my Bible and sat it on my lap. After catching my breath, I prayed, "Lord, I may not be able to take in your Word, but I can still trust your Word." Suddenly I had a peace that surpassed all understanding.

The problem with many today is not that they cannot take in God's Word but that they will not trust God's Word. And better than taking in God's Word and stopping there, is taking in God's Word and trusting God's Word. Civil War General Robert E. Lee said, "In all my perplexities and distresses, the Bible has never failed to give me light and strength."

Fortunately, the medicine I was on only affected my short-term memory. Though I could not remember what I had just read, I could remember what I had read over the years. Those verses I had known since childhood began flooding into my mind. Passages like Romans 8:28, "And we know that all things work together for good to those who love God, to those who are the called according to His purpose." And Philippians 4:13, "I can do all things through Christ who strengthens me." And Hebrews 13:5, "I will never leave you nor forsake you." And Jeremiah 29:11, "For I know the thoughts that

I think toward you, says the LORD, thoughts of peace and not of evil, to give you a future and a hope."

Let me ask you a question. If your short-term memory was removed, would you still be able to feed upon God's Word? Let me ask it another way. Have you hid enough of God's Word in your heart and mind to survive a short-term memory loss? You say, "Ernest, I don't know the Word of God." Whose fault is that? You will never get to know God well enough to trust God without spending time in his Word. God has something to say to you, and you are missing it. God's Word is trustworthy. He has given you some bedrock promises within his Word! Take them in and trust them. Especially when you find yourself in the valley of confusion.

The next promise that comforted Habakkuk was that God will punish every sin. Though it appeared that God was not going to punish the sins of his people, five times in chapter 2 God says "woe," which is a pronouncement of judgment. "Woe to him who increases what is not his—how long?" (v. 6).

"Woe to him who covets evil gain for his house, that he may set his nest on high" (v. 9). "Woe to him who builds a town with bloodshed, who establishes a city by iniquity!" (v. 12). "Woe to him who gives drink to his neighbor, pressing him to your bottle" (v. 15). "Woe to him who says to wood, 'Awake!' To silent stone, 'Arise! It shall teach!' Behold, it is overlaid with gold and silver, yet in it there is no breath at all" (v. 19).

God knows about every sin, and he is going to judge them, including yours! It may appear that the world is getting by with their sin, but not for long. Remember, just because you are involved in sins and God has seemingly let it slide does not mean that God will let it slide forever! You can be grateful that God is slow to wrath, but one of these days every unconfessed, unforgiven sin will be judged. Thank God for the promise of I John 1:9, "If we confess our sins, He is faithful and just to forgive us our sins and to cleanse us from all unrighteousness."

Habakkuk also found comfort in knowing that God will ultimately be victorious. "For the earth will be filled with the knowledge of the glory of the LORD, as the waters cover the sea" (2:14).

Here is how the apostle Paul said it in Philippians 2:10–11, "That at the name of Jesus every knee should bow, of those in heaven, and of those on earth, and of those under the earth, and that every tongue should confess that Jesus Christ is Lord, to the glory of God the Father."

How comforting and reassuring to know that while you are in the valley of confusion, King Jesus continues ruling and reigning! Regardless of the depth and width of your valley, Jesus remains on the throne. He was ruling yesterday. He is ruling today. And he will be ruling tomorrow. Praise his name!

THE PRAYER THAT CHANGED HIM

I don't know a better time to pray than when confusion strikes. There were many nights throughout my treatments when I would wake up praying. I would pray myself to sleep and then pick up where I left off when I woke up in the middle of the night. I remember one night waking up in tears. I rolled over to face my wife and said, "Julie, pray for me." There is nothing like a godly, praying spouse.

In Habakkuk 3, we get to listen in on this man's prayer. His prayer is full of praise and thanksgiving. Take a few minutes to read through it slowly. Here is a man who had learned to offer praise to God, though he was confused and frustrated. Here is a man who had learned to trust God. He had learned what the apostle Paul would record many years later when he said, "Rejoice in the Lord always. Again I will say, rejoice!" (Phil. 4:4).

Let me take you to the conclusion of his prayer. In wrapping up his prayer, we hear how his prayer changed the direction of his focus. "Though the fig tree may not blossom, nor fruit be on the vines; though the labor of the olive may fail, and the fields yield no food; though the flock be cut off from the fold, and there be no herd in the stalls—yet I will rejoice in the LORD, I will joy in the God of my salvation. The LORD God is my strength; He will make my feet like deer's feet, and He will make me walk on my high hills" (Hab. 3:17–19).

What happened to Habakkuk happens to us all. He got his focus on his circumstances and off of God. But as he began praying, his focus changed. Now he has his focus off of his circumstances and back on God. He is no longer pouting; he is praising. You cannot pout and praise at the same time. You cannot gripe and glorify God at the same time. Valley or no valley, God desires and delights in the praises of his children. He not only desires and delights in our praises, he honors them.

Praise is a wonderful medicine to try when you find yourself in the valley of confusion. As difficult as it is to comprehend, I experienced an incredible peace as I offered praise to God throughout my battle with cancer. The same kind of peace that Habakkuk experienced as his prayer changed his focus. Now, rather than shouting at God, he is offering praise to God. Now he is saying, "Yet I will rejoice in the LORD, I will joy in the God of my salvation. The LORD God is my strength" (vv. 18–19). Do you hear the difference? Learn this: praise is the secret to experiencing peace in the valley.

Are you in the valley of confusion today? Embrace God. Trust him. Praise him. Ron Dunn was correct when he said, "I have been to the bottom, and I'm here to tell you it's solid." And from one who has been there, it is!

The Valley of
CORRECTION

Jonah 1–2

But Jonah arose to flee to Tarshish from the presence of the
LORD. He went down to Joppa, and found a ship going to
Tarshish; so he paid the fare, and went down into it, to go
with them to Tarshish from the presence of the LORD.

Jonah 1:3

I HOPE BY NOW THAT YOU ARE BEGINNING to understand there is victory in the valleys. Spiritual victory. Personal victory. Physical victory. Valleys are where you learn to trust and depend on God. That was what the apostle Paul was saying in Romans 8:28, "And we know that all things [including valleys] work together for good to those who love God, to those who are the called according to His purpose."

Life's valleys will turn you into either a victim or a victor, depending on your response. Know this: *God is pulling for you in every valley.* He longs to see you experience victory through every battle and lives to make intercession for you. Knowing that Jesus was praying for me during my deepest valley gave me peace and assurance. And you can know this today: *Jesus is praying for you.*

We have discovered so far that God allows some valleys for perfecting, that is, to make us more like him. That is what happened to
Joseph. God used that valley in Joseph's life to mature and mold him
to become a mighty man of God.

Now let me ask you a question about Joseph: Was it his personal
sin that caused his valley? No, he was not in that valley because
he did something wrong but because he did something right. What
others meant for evil, God meant for good.

Sometimes God uses valleys for perfecting. Other times though,
he uses valleys for instructing. That is what happened to Jesus' disciples. He sent them into a storm on the Sea of Galilee to teach them
something. And what he taught them out on the sea they would have
never learned back on the shore.

And like Joseph, they found themselves in a valley because they
obeyed the Word of God. Their obedience to Jesus landed them in
the middle of a storm! Some valleys are used in our life for perfecting while other valleys are used for instructing. But there are other
times when God uses valleys in our life for correcting. In other
words, God uses valleys to get you back in step with him after you
have rebelled against him. That is what happened to the Old
Testament prophet named Jonah. God told Jonah to go, and he said
no and ended up in a whale of a mess.

Before we look at what happened to Jonah, let me settle the issue
of the validity of his valley. I believe that Jonah was a real person
who rebelled against God and was literally tossed into the sea, then
swallowed by a real fish, then was spit out on the beach. Literally!
And here's why: the Bible tells me so.

Those who call into question what happened to Jonah in his rebellion must also call into question what happened to Jesus in his resurrection. Here is what Jesus said in Matthew 12:40: "For as Jonah was three days and three nights in the belly of the great fish, so will the Son of Man be three days and three nights in the heart of the earth." God performed a miracle in rescuing the prophet Jonah just as he performed a miracle in resurrecting his only begotten Son, the Lord Jesus Christ.

If what the Bible says about Jonah is not true, then what the Bible says about Jesus is not true. Jesus illustrated his death, burial, and resurrection by pointing to what happened to Jonah!

Sometimes it is possible to choose a valley over a mountaintop. For example, Jesus chose a valley by becoming sin. And when you choose sin, valleys are sure to follow. That is what happened to the prophet Jonah. His sin landed him in the valley of the deep blue sea.

Joseph found himself in a valley because of obedience. Jonah, on the other hand, found himself in a valley because of disobedience. And yet God used both valleys to bring victory into their lives. God used the disciples' valley for instructing. He used Joseph's valley for perfecting, and he used Jonah's valley for correcting.

You can know that rebellion against God will always land you in the valley of correction, and here is why: to draw you back to him. Back into fellowship with him. Back into his loving and caring arms. Back to worshipping him. Do you see it? There is victory even in the valley of correction.

How did it happen in Jonah's life? Jonah was confronted with several things.

THE WORD OF THE LORD

The first thing the book of Jonah tells us is that "the word of the LORD" was delivered to Jonah. Jonah 1:1 says, "Now the word of the LORD came to Jonah the son of Amittai." We are not told how the word of the LORD was delivered, only that it was delivered. However it was delivered, we know it was received. Jonah got it. He heard God's word loud and clear.

The same is true today. God speaks loud and clear on every page of his Word and regarding every issue of life. Don't think that today God is silent. He is still speaking, and his Word never changes. The question is not whether God is speaking but whether you are listening.

What did God say to Jonah? We read in verse 2, "Arise, go to Nineveh, that great city, and cry out against it; for their wickedness has come up before Me." Simple and plain. God instructed this prophet to get up and get going to the godless city of Nineveh, to preach the good news of salvation and forgiveness.

Were the Ninevites a wicked people? Yes. Were they despised by the Israelites? Yes. Was this prophet willing to go? No. Not only was the word of the Lord delivered; it was disobeyed. God told Jonah to go, and he said no.

"But Jonah arose to flee to Tarshish from the presence of the LORD. He went down to Joppa, and found a ship going to Tarshish; so he paid the fare, and went down into it, to go with them to Tarshish from the presence of the LORD" (v. 3). Jonah decided that day to disobey the word of God. He was not going to Nineveh. He was not going to preach salvation to those godless Ninevites.

He dug in his heels and said, "I'm not going. I resign from being a prophet."

Now let me ask you a question: What is the difference in Jonah's disobedience and your disobedience? None. Same God. Same word. Same disobedience.

Let me ask you another question: If Jonah's disobedience landed him in the valley of correction, why would your disobedience not land you in the same valley? Do you think God responds differently to disobedience today? The answer is a resounding no! Whenever you disobey the Word and will of God, you have taken a step toward the valley of correction.

It took several days for me to overcome the shock of hearing that I had throat cancer. As the reality of my illness began to sink in, I began to take a personal inventory. *Was this cancer a result of my sin? Have I disobeyed God? Am I living in rebellion against God? And if so, what sin? What disobedience? What rebellion?*

I cried out, "Lord, if this cancer is due to sin, point it out, and I will ask you to root it out. I will repent. I will come clean. If this is the result of my disobedience to you, show me. If there is any rebellion within me, tell me. I will turn back to you."

Every crisis is an opportunity to take a personal inventory, making sure things are right between you and God. Perhaps your inventory, like mine, will reveal a growing relationship with God. On the other hand, it may reveal, like Jonah, a rebellion against God. Jonah tried to run from the presence of God.

You may be running from God today. You may be running from salvation. You may be running from repentance. You may be running from reconciliation. Do you realize the direction you are headed?

The same direction Jonah was headed: Down to Joppa, down into the ship. Down. Down. Down. And to tell you how good God is, he is waiting for you in the valley of correction. Ready to restore you. Ready to reuse you. You see, there is victory in the valleys.

The Wind from the Lord

"But the LORD sent out a great wind on the sea, and there was a mighty tempest on the sea, so that the ship was about to be broken up" (Jonah 1:4). Now the wind from the Lord caused several things. To begin with, the wind caused a storm. To tell you how severe the storm was, verse 5 tells us that "the mariners were afraid; and every man cried out to his god." These men were professionals. They had spent a lot of time out on the sea. That was their job. They had seen lots of storms. But when they saw this storm, they were afraid.

Who sent this storm? God sent it, that's who. You are reading about a God-sent storm to a God-called man. You say, "If God really loved Jonah, he would never have put him in that kind of danger." God did not send that storm because he didn't love Jonah; he sent it because he loved Jonah.

The wind not only caused a storm; it caused a sleep. "But Jonah had gone down into the lowest parts of the ship, had lain down, and was fast asleep. So the captain came to him, and said to him, 'What do you mean, sleeper? Arise, call on your God; perhaps your God will consider us, so that we may not perish'" (Jonah 1:5–6).

The devil is a master at lulling God's children to sleep in their rebellion. Jonah was not only sleeping physically; he was sleeping spiritually. God sent a storm to wake him up out of his rebellion.

Perhaps God is attempting to wake you up. Like Jonah, you're trying to run from the presence of God. You are headed in the same direction that Jonah was headed: down, down, down. No wonder you are in the valley of correction. But remember, it was your choice.

Not only did the wind from the Lord cause a storm and a sleep; it also caused a struggle.

> And they said to one another, "Come, let us cast lots, that we may know for whose cause this trouble has come upon us." So they cast lots, and the lot fell on Jonah. Then they said to him, "Please tell us! For whose cause is this trouble upon us? What is your occupation? And where do you come from? What is your country? And of what people are you?" And he said to them, "I am a Hebrew; and I fear the LORD, the God of heaven, who made the sea and the dry land." Then the men were exceedingly afraid, and said to him, "Why have you done this?" For the men knew that he fled from the presence of the LORD, because he had told them (Jonah 1:7–10).

Don't ever believe the lie that your sin only affects you! Satan whispers, "Go ahead. Nobody else will ever find out. You won't hurt anybody." And then we give in to the temptation, and Satan begins laughing because we've believed the lie again.

You can believe that sin always affects others, often those we love the most. Jonah's sin affected these strangers, and even those godless mariners realized it. They cried out, "Why have you done this?"

You can count on struggles in the valley of correction. Struggles in your marriage. Struggles with your children. Struggles in your business. Physical struggles. Spiritual struggles. Emotional struggles.

Do yourself and those around you a favor: repent and return to God. Experience the victory in the valley of correction.

THE WILL OF THE LORD

"Now the LORD had prepared a great fish to swallow Jonah. And Jonah was in the belly of the fish three days and three nights" (Jonah 1:17). How was the will of the Lord accomplished in the life of this backslidden prophet? To begin with, this backslidden prophet was repentant.

"So they picked up Jonah and threw him into the sea, and the sea ceased from its raging" (Jonah 1:15). You can believe that when Jonah hit the water, and it suddenly calmed down, he knew that his running from God was indeed the cause of the storm. "Then the men feared the LORD exceedingly, and offered a sacrifice to the LORD and took vows" (v. 16). I'm sure they did make vows, like, never again traveling with a backslidden prophet. By the way, it's interesting how these mariners turned to the Lord after the backslidden prophet turned back to God.

What did Jonah do next? He stopped fighting and started surrendering. The moment he repented, calmness came. The moment he repented, peace came and the storm ceased. You say, "How do you know that Jonah repented?" To begin with, the storm stopped and the praying started! He concluded his prayer, "But I will sacrifice to You with the voice of thanksgiving; I will pay what I have vowed. Salvation is of the LORD" (2:9).

The will of the Lord was accomplished. Yes, Jonah was repentant, and then he was rescued. "Now the LORD had prepared a great fish to swallow Jonah. And Jonah was in the belly of the fish three days and three nights" (1:17). Rescued by a great fish. God rescued this prophet not only for his good but for the good of the Ninevites. God rescued Jonah so that others might be saved. In the same way God resurrected Jesus so that the world might be saved.

Don't miss this. Jonah first rebelled against the word of God. After he rebelled he then repented. After he repented he was rescued. He was rescued in order to be restored. He was restored in order to be released: "So the LORD spoke to the fish, and it vomited Jonah onto dry land" (2:10). He was released in order to be reused: "And Jonah began to enter the city on the first day's walk. Then he cried out and said, 'Yet forty days, and Nineveh shall be overthrown!' So the people of Nineveh believed God, proclaimed a fast, and put on sackcloth, from the greatest to the least of them. . . . Then God saw their works, that they turned from their evil way; and God relented from the disaster that He had said He would bring upon them, and He did not do it" (3:4–5, 10).

Do you see the sequence? Rebelled. Repented. Rescued. Restored. Released. Reused. Jonah landed in the valley of correction by his own choosing. But just as he chose to rebel, he chose to repent. And through his repentance, God restored him and then reused him. There is victory through the valleys, including the valley of correction.

The Valley of
SICKNESS

James 5:13–16

Is anyone among you sick? Let him call for the elders of the
church, and let them pray over him, anointing him with oil in
the name of the Lord. And the prayer of faith will save the
sick, and the Lord will raise him up.

James 5:14–15

IF YOU LIVE LONG ENOUGH, you will spend some time in the valley
of sickness. For me the valley of sickness drove me to my knees and
into God's Word. But for many people today, the valley of sickness
drives them halfway around the world to get in touch with those who
claim to have the gift of healing. The popular teaching that your
sickness can simply be prayed away is often sought and practiced
when sickness strikes. Others will tell you that when you are sick, you
are not really sick at all. It is all in your head. If you convince yourself that you are not sick, then you won't be.

With so many options, where do you turn? Where do you go?
Whom do you seek? When you find yourself in the valley of sickness, what do you do? If you can settle those questions while you are

healthy, when sickness strikes, you won't have to spend valuable time and energy trying to decide where to turn. It is like preparing for a tornado. If you wait until the tornado strikes, you are more likely to panic and make poor decisions. But if you have already decided where the safest place is to go, all you have to do when the tornado comes is to head to that safe place. The only decision you have to make is how to get there fast.

Sickness is the same way. When I found myself in the valley of sickness, there was no decision to make regarding where I would turn. That decision was predetermined. I would turn to prayer and to the promises of God. These two life-savers gave me strength, hope, and peace as I journeyed through the valley of sickness.

In concluding this book, I want to turn to the New Testament book of James. The Holy Spirit, through pastor James, gives us some practical and personal help when it comes to sickness. I must tell you that though I had predetermined my course of action—prayer and standing on God's promises—there were some surprises along the way. Even after six years since my valley of sickness, I still shake my head in amazement and wonder.

ENGAGE IN PRAYER

James says: "Is anyone among you suffering? Let him pray. . . . Is anyone among you sick? Let him call for the elders of the church, and let them pray over him. . . . And the prayer of faith will save the sick. . . . And pray for one another, that you may be healed. The effective, fervent prayer of a righteous man avails much. . . . He prayed earnestly. . . . And he prayed again" (James 5:13–18).

Seven times in six verses James tells us that sickness is a summons to pray. Pray for what? I suppose James figured that you would know what to pray for. When I got sick, nobody had to sit me down and say, "Now Ernest, you need to pray for this and pray for that." No, I knew what to pray for. I prayed for healing. I prayed for wisdom. I prayed for strength. I prayed for God to lead me to the best physicians. Then I prayed for each of them individually. I prayed for more grace. I prayed for my family. I prayed for my church. I prayed when I woke up in the mornings. I prayed in the afternoons. I prayed during radiation treatments. I prayed myself to sleep.

Engage in prayer. I read years ago that prayer can do anything God can do, and God can do anything. No wonder James says to engage in prayer when sickness strikes.

God says, "Call upon Me in the day of trouble; I will deliver you, and you shall glorify Me" (Ps. 50:15). Every sickness is a call to prayer. Every setback is a summons to prayer.

In fact, in verse 13 where James says, "Let him pray," he uses a present tense verb in the Greek language. It could be translated, "Let him pray and keep on praying." Don't think that your praying is complete once it is offered! In fact, Paul says the same thing in I Thessalonians 5:17, "Pray without ceasing" (literally, "Pray and keep on praying without ceasing").

Not only is it a present tense verb; it is in the imperative. In other words, it is a command. God commands the sick to pray and keep on praying. You have been commanded by Almighty God to pray and keep on praying. Somebody asks, "How long do I pray?" Until you get an answer. Engage in prayer and keep on engaging in prayer until you hear from heaven!

ENLIST OTHERS TO PRAY

Not only are you to engage in prayer; you are to enlist others to pray. There are several aspects to this enlistment. It begins with calling. "Is anyone among you sick? Let him call . . ." (James 5:14). When you get sick, pick up the phone, get on your e-mail address book, and start calling on people to pray for you. That's right, you are to take the initiative. Don't wait around for somebody to call you; you call them.

You say, "That's not my place to call. They ought to call me." I don't know where you got that, but you did not get it from the Word of God. It is your place to call. God says so. In fact, when James says, "Let him call," he once again uses the imperative. Not only are you to call, you are commanded by God to call. And if that is not enough, you are not only commanded to call, you are commanded to call and keep on calling (present tense).

Whom do you call? James says to call "the elders of the church." Who are the "elders of the church"? Don't get the idea that the elders are the senior adults in the church. The elders may be among the senior adults, but not necessarily. The elders in your church may be in their twenties or thirties.

The Greek word translated "elders" is used interchangeably throughout the New Testament with the words *pastor* and *bishop*. It refers to the spiritual leaders in the church. They could include the pastor, a deacon, a staff member, a Sunday school teacher, a Bible study leader, and anyone else in a place of spiritual leadership.

When you find yourself in the valley of sickness, don't sneak off to the hospital without enlisting the spiritual leaders in your church to pray and then complain that nobody called to check on you. It is your responsibility to call and enlist others to pray for you.

Did you notice whose prayer has real power? "The effective, fervent prayer of a righteous man avails much" (v. 16). When I became sick, I not only enlisted the elders to pray; I enlisted the righteous to pray. Those who are righteous, those who are in right standing with God, those who walk with God and serve God and strive to honor God, have a prayer life like no other. James says that their prayer "avails" or accomplishes much.

Enlisting others to pray involves calling. It also involves cooperation, cooperating with God's laws of healing. "Is anyone among you sick? Let him call for the elders of the church, and let them pray over him, anointing him with oil in the name of the Lord" (James 5:14). What is James suggesting? Is anointing with oil to be included with the prayers of the elders?

As you can imagine, there are several ideas behind "anointing with oil." Two distinct words in the Greek New Testament are translated *anoint.* One is a sacred use while the other is a secular use. An example of the sacred use is found in Acts 10:38: "How God anointed [*chrio*] Jesus of Nazareth with the Holy Spirit and with power." Here is the sacred use of the word *anoint.* It is used of anointing kings and as a symbol of the Holy Spirit. This is not the word James uses when he says, "anointing him with oil." James uses the secular word (*aleipho*), which means "to grease down, to massage, to rub into the skin."

This word was used to describe the athletes of Greece when they would have their bodies rubbed with oil to relax them. The anointing James is talking about is not the anointing for religious ceremony. He is talking about anointing in the secular sense to relieve physical suffering. Olive oil was used as a medical commodity in the first century to relieve suffering and pain and is still used today.

By the way, the Greek language suggests that the anointing should take place *before* the praying. Verse 14 could be translated, "Let them pray over him having anointed him with oil." First comes anointing, then comes praying. In other words, seek the best medical care available first and then pray.

I was discussing recently with Jerry Vines, the senior pastor of the First Baptist Church of Jacksonville, Florida, about biblical anointing and how it was applied to me during my sickness. He made an interesting observation. He said, "Ernest, you really received two kinds of anointing. First, you were anointed twice with oil, and then you were anointed forty-four times with radiation."

Before traveling to Houston to seek treatments at M. D. Anderson Cancer Center, my local ear, nose, and throat specialist had removed my right tonsil, the main source of the cancer. (By the way, I would suggest having a tonsillectomy when you are young. It took days of recovery before I could begin swallowing food again.)

By this time word was out in our community about my cancer, surgery, and plans to go to Houston for treatments. One afternoon while I was recovering from the tonsillectomy, our doorbell rang. I was somewhat drowsy due to medication, but I overheard my wife talking to a man at the front door. Moments later this stranger was squatting beside my recliner introducing himself to me.

He began telling me who he was. He told me about his love for Jesus and that he had heard about my cancer. He then asked me something I had never been asked before: "Would you mind if I anointed you with oil?"

I was thinking, *How in the world did he get in here? Doesn't he know that I am a conservative, Bible-believing Baptist preacher? And if he does know it, why is he beside my chair asking permission to anoint me with oil?*

I was stunned! As I looked into his eyes, I saw a man of compassion who believed he was on a mission from God. I sensed his sincerity, though I didn't agree with his interpretation of James 5:14. I remember thinking, *Here I sit recovering from a painful tonsillectomy, wondering if I am going to live or die, not sure what to do next, and I'm going to tell this brother in Christ that he cannot anoint me with oil?*

I looked at him and said, "Yes, you may." He then pulled out a small vile of oil, opened it, and poured a small amount of oil on the crown of my head. Even as I write this, I can still smell it. Next, this brother in Christ asked permission to pray. Permission was granted, and afterwards, he walked out of my house. I had never seen him prior to that event, nor have I ever heard from him since.

I was born in Houston, Texas. In fact, often I would drive past the hospital where I was born on the way to M. D. Anderson for radiation treatments. The first time we rode past, I thought, *Isn't this great? I'm going to die a few blocks from where I was born!*

Our family left Houston in 1961, when I was four years old, to move to Dallas. One weekend during my treatments, my parents and my only sister and her husband came for a visit. Knowing they were coming, I felt a sudden urge for our family to return to the house we left thirty-six years ago. We drove to the little house on Glenmore Street that we once called home.

During the thirty-minute ride, we reminisced about neighborhood friends, trying to remember their names. My sister, who is three years older, remembered more than I did. When we arrived, my father walked up to the porch and knocked on the door. The front door opened, and a two-minute conversation took place. He walked back to the car and said, "I told the man we used to live here and asked if we could come in. He said that we could." My father, mother, sister, and I walked into the same den that the four of us left thirty-six years ago. It seemed like a dream.

After a short tour (it was extremely small), my father explained to the owner why we were there. He explained that I had throat cancer and was taking treatments at M. D. Anderson Cancer Center and that I was a Baptist pastor. We learned that this man's parents bought the house from us in 1961, and now he was living there.

After talking with him a few more minutes, he looked at me in the same way that my visitor back in Odessa looked and said, "Would you mind if I prayed and anointed you before you leave?"

I thought, *He must have a first cousin living in Odessa.* By this time, I had experience in this anointing thing. With less hesitation than before, I said, "Yes, you may." There in our kitchen, sitting around a table, in the home we left thirty-six years ago, this stranger took a small portion of oil, poured it on the crown of my head, and began to pray.

At the conclusion of his prayer, I stood up, and he looked me in the eyes and said, "You will be healed."

I remember thinking, *I pray that you're right.* That was the first and last time I ever laid eyes on him.

What do you do when you find yourself in the valley of sickness? First, engage in prayer. Second, enlist others to pray. And in doing so there is calling and cooperation. Cooperate with God's laws of healing. Seek out the best medical care you can find . . . and pray.

Next comes cleansing. "And the prayer of faith will save the sick, and the Lord will raise him up. And if he has committed sins, he will be forgiven" (James 5:15). I don't know a better healing than forgiveness. Being right with God and man has a way of healing a lot of wounds.

My battle with throat cancer branded two words on my mind that I want to pass along to you: *attentive* and *aggressive.* You need to stay attentive to your body. Annual physicals and checkups should be a part of your routine, especially after you turn forty years old. Self-examinations should be done periodically. Watch for any changes that occur on your body, especially moles. Be attentive to your body.

Along with being attentive, be aggressive. When you find something not normal or something that is new, immediately seek a physician. Don't put it off. Be attentive. Be aggressive.

Do I believe in healing? Of course I believe in healing, and I'll tell you why: because I believe God. God says in Exodus 15:26, "For I am the LORD who heals you."

Does God always heal? No. God has healed. God can heal. God will heal. But God is not obligated always to heal. When it comes to healing, this one thing I know: there is no healing except divine healing.

Will God heal Ernest Easley if his cancer returns? Perhaps, if it will bring him the most glory, he will. If healing will be for my good, he will. Will I pray for healing the next time I get sick? Absolutely. Will I trust him with the outcome? Absolutely. Is there really victory through the valleys? What do you think?

CONCLUSION

VICTORY COMES THROUGH THE VALLEYS, though it is often difficult to realize when you are there. Every valley has value. God teaches us things in the valleys that we would never learn on the mountaintops.

When we spend time in the valleys, we learn more about truth and trust—the truth of God's Word. It's one thing to read God's Word and believe God's Word; it's another thing to live God's Word.

For instance, I knew what Paul said in 2 Corinthians 12:9 in quoting the Lord Jesus: "My grace is sufficient for you, for My strength is made perfect in weakness." Now I knew a lot about God's grace being sufficient for saving me, but I knew little about God's grace being sufficient for sustaining me. That is, until I found myself fighting for my life. Until I found myself in a very deep valley. Had it not been for that valley, I still wouldn't know that much about God's sustaining grace.

Now having experienced God's sustaining grace through that valley, I love him more, praise him more, and trust him more. It is not that I did not love him and praise him and trust him prior to my valley, but the valley brought my love, praise, and trust to a different level.

Those valleys not only teach us about the truth of God's Word. We also learn while there about trusting God's Word. Trust may be established when all is well, but trust is built when all is wrong. When I invited the Lord Jesus into my heart to save me and to be my Lord, trust was established. That is when I began trusting him to save and forgive me. Having established that trust with God, he now wants that trust to be built, to be strengthened. Trust is built and strengthened through struggles and hardships. There is no other way. No wonder Paul said in Philippians 4:4, "Rejoice in the Lord always. Again I will say, rejoice."

If anybody understood how trust was built, it was the apostle Paul. His trust in God's Word grew through hardships, and so does ours. That's why you can rejoice today in your valley. That's why you can praise your way through every valley. The valley life leads to the victorious life.

You can rejoice knowing that through the valleys you learn the truth of God's Word and to trust God's Word. Is it easy? Absolutely not. Nobody ever said it was. In fact, it may be the hardest thing you ever experience and endure. Is it worth it? Absolutely.

When valleys come, we wonder not only how they will turn out but how long they will last. Just as valleys begin they eventually end, with surprises along the way. The psalmist tells us, "Weeping may endure for a night, but joy comes in the morning" (Ps. 30:5).

You may be experiencing a dark valley these days, full of weeping. There were several nights I went to sleep weeping and woke up weeping. Let me remind you that morning is coming and, with it, joy, the kind of joy that only the presence of God can produce.

In the meantime, trust him. Know that God has not forsaken you (Heb. 13:5). Know that he is a present help in times of trouble (Ps. 46:1). Know that you can trust the Lord forever, for the Lord is everlasting strength (Isa. 26:4). Know that you need not fear, for God says, "Fear not, for I am with you; be not dismayed, for I am your God. I will strengthen you, yes, I will help you, I will uphold you with My righteous right hand" (Isa. 41:10).

"Weeping may endure for a night, but joy comes in the morning" (Ps. 30:5).